How to End Anxiety

*Get Relief from Anxiety, Depression and
Overcoming Panic Attacks in Your
Relationships Through Meditation Practice*

Caroline Kirkman

Table of Contents

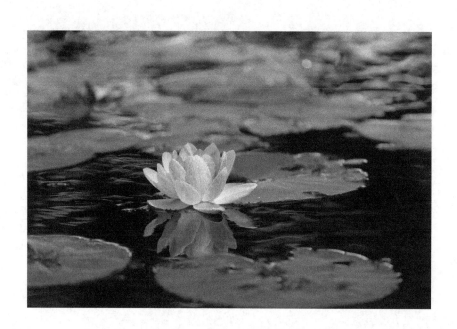

Introduction

Everyone has been anxious at one point or another in their lives. It is a common feeling. Maybe you have experienced your heart racing before a big presentation, or you sweating more than usual on a first date. Anxiety is a natural part of life that helps people to be aware of potentially scary or dangerous situations. In fact, without it, people might not have made it this far in the evolutionary journey. Some people, however, struggle with anxiety on a regular basis and not just in stressful or scary moments. These people can sometimes handle their symptoms on their own and might find effective ways to cope, but sometimes they cannot handle it alone and have to seek help. This usually occurs in people who are diagnosed with an anxiety disorder.

What is Anxiety?

Anxiety involves intense feelings of dread or fear that can be related to a particular activity or situation. In the caveman days, it was the brain's mechanism to keep people aware of their surroundings, but today, people are much less likely to be attacked by wild animals in their day-to-day life. In some people this lack of direct danger results in free-floating anxiety about life, or generalized anxiety, because their brain is unable to switch out of its fight-or-flight mode. Anxiety can go so far as disrupting a person's life by making them unable to perform basic tasks or uninterested in things they used to enjoy because they are so afraid of feeling anxious.

Some people experience anxiety to such an extreme that they start experiencing panic attacks. These are intense anxiety episodes that come on suddenly and usually last around 10 to 30 minutes. They trigger an array of physical symptoms that make a person feel like they are having a heart attack or having trouble breathing. Just like with anxiety, some people might experience a panic attack every now and then and be able to ride it out and continue with normal life, but others are plagued by them. Someone who frequently experiences panic attacks might be diagnosed with panic disorder and need assistance to get their anxiety under control.

How to Heal

There are a wide range of options and therapies for people who suffer from anxiety and panic attacks. Most of these treatments include the person seeking out a mental health professional who can assist them with controlling their thoughts and behaviors to start slowly erasing anxiety from their minds and lives. Typically, these doctors will use cognitive behavioral therapy, which focuses on altering the person's thoughts and behaviors so they begin to realize on their own that their fears are not real threats.

Finding the right type of therapy for a person, though, depends on their specific needs.

Other ways people can manage their anxious feelings on their own include meditative practices such as mindfulness and yoga. Meditation has a wide variety of benefits for both mental and physical health and can help people with anxiety clear their mind of negative thoughts and have a moment of peace during the day.

Chapter 1: What is Anxiety?

Anxiety is a natural response to fear or danger and can keep people safe in certain situations. Some people, however, experience anxiety more severely than others. This can lead to anxiety disorders, which can cause people to make major changes in their lives and habits to avoid situations or places that they believe cause them anxiety. If symptoms are persistent, a person might even be diagnosed with an anxiety disorder and recommended to seek treatment. Anxiety disorders can present themselves in a variety of ways; panic attacks, social anxiety, phobias, and separation anxiety to name a few.

A person might experience a host of physical symptoms with their anxiety, which can sometimes make it seem worse. Besides the unhealthy negative thoughts that are racing through their brain, they might also feel their heart racing, their temperature rising, or their breathing becoming shallower. These are all typical fight-or-flight responses that are triggered by anxiety to encourage a person to avoid the situation because the brain is perceiving it as a threat. It can be difficult for people to ignore thoughts of fear and dread when their body is pitching in and seemingly confirming them.

People experience anxiety for many different reasons, usually depending on their own life experiences and how their past has affected them. Some people have triggers for their anxiety, such as social situations or being separated from somewhere they feel is a safe space. Others feel anxiety in relation to nothing in particular but are constantly plagued with thoughts of fear and danger throughout the day. It can be difficult to deal with anxious feelings on a daily basis, but there are some things people can do to help ease the tension. This chapter discusses the psychology of anxiety, common symptoms, potential triggers, and ways to find relief.

Anxiety Explained

Anxiety can be difficult for people to recognize when they are first experiencing it. Most people, in fact, might mistake it for a physical health problem due to the symptoms that accompany it. At its core, anxiety is a response to stress. It makes people feel scared or worried about certain situations for a variety of reasons. Some people might be worried that others will judge them for how they act or speak, others might be afraid that some harm will come to them if they put themselves in a certain situation. These feelings are not all abnormal, however. Some common anxiety-inducing situations include a child's first day of school, an initial job interview, or someone's wedding day. These experiences can all cause anxiety due to the uncertainty of the situation and might cause a person to start thinking about worst-case scenarios.

All of these feelings are part of anxiety because it was the evolutionary way of keeping people safe when their environment was inherently dangerous. The heightening of senses and increased heart rate prepares the body to run or fight if presented with danger, which could have meant life or death in prehistoric times. Today, however, people are not faced with imminent death on a daily basis, but their brain might not know how to adjust itself to the safety of modern life. It can still trigger anxious feelings if it is threatened to encourage a person to flee the situation, even if the reasons are not rational.

Some people experience anxiety to an extreme degree and can feel like their negative thoughts are unrelenting. For someone with this level of anxiety, quieting their mind and finding any kind of relief can be especially difficult and might even seem impossible. If a person suffers from anxiety of this intensity for an extended period of time, they might fit the criteria for an anxiety disorder. Typically, to qualify for a disorder diagnosis, a person has to experience symptoms for longer than six months or the symptoms need to be interfering with their daily life.

There are a variety of anxiety disorders that are all defined by how the anxiety affects someone or what causes anxious feelings. Each person is different, even though they might experience similar symptoms of anxiety, and the way their anxiety affects them can make a big difference in a diagnosis. Among these disorders is a plethora of negative side effects caused by the increased levels of stress and constant negative thoughts. Some people have trouble sleeping at night, have trouble concentrating during the day, find interacting with others especially difficult, or are too afraid to leave their own homes.

Some common anxiety disorders include panic disorder, phobias, social anxiety disorder, and separation anxiety. Obsessive-compulsive disorder is no longer considered an anxiety disorder, but people diagnosed with it often experience severe anxiety as one of their symptoms. Each of these common disorders associate anxiety with a particular object, situation, or action. These disorders can severely affect a person's life by making them unable to perform daily tasks or prevent them from enjoying their hobbies. For example, someone with agoraphobia—fear of crowds—may become so debilitated by fear that they refuse to leave their home.

The symptoms of anxiety are not necessarily universal and can vary greatly from person to person. Sometimes the reason a person has anxiety can determine their symptoms, as well. For example, someone who has anxiety because they think they are in danger might feel a pounding heart because their body wants to escape. Another person, however, who is dreading a social interaction, might experience an upset stomach due to the increased stress. Symptoms can range from gastrointestinal issues to cardiovascular discomfort, headaches, and in extreme cases even vomiting if stress builds up enough with the anxiety.

At the onset of symptoms, some people may suddenly feel like they are no longer in control of their body. This can often increase feelings of anxiety because they may not feel like the dread or physical symptoms will ever subside. Sometimes this out of control feeling can even lead to panic attacks. Other startling symptoms can include nightmares or constantly recalling painful thoughts or memories. These can also contribute to increased stress and anxiety because a person might feel like they cannot escape their own negative thoughts or what might seem to be an inevitably painful outcome of an event.

In people with generalized anxiety, it is more common to worry about things because of a past experience. For example, if a child's parent forgot them in a grocery store for an extended time, that child might then develop a fear of grocery stores and feel unsafe when they go to one. This could potentially carry on into adulthood, even if the person doesn't remember the event that instigated their anxiety. Common symptoms of this type of anxiety usually present themselves when a person is in a certain situation or sometimes if they merely consider putting themselves in the trigger situation. These people often experience a racing heart, shortness of breath or rapid breathing, restlessness, trouble focusing, and a slew of other symptoms.

Anxiety can even affect a person's stomach function, causing gas, constipation, or diarrhea when it flares up. This can also contribute to more severe anxiety in a person because they may become fixated on their stomach problems and convinced that if they are in a social situation they might have a problem they cannot get away to handle. Some people can experience this discomfort even at the thought of doing something that gives them anxiety. This is why it can be particularly difficult for people to overcome their anxiety. If even the thought of doing something makes them feel physically ill, it can be difficult to convince themselves that actually doing it won't be painful.

When people experience these intense physical symptoms in relation to their anxiety, it can often cause them to start avoiding things, situations, or people that they believe will trigger their negative feelings. Although this might seem like an effective coping mechanism to those with anxiety, it can actually severely limit their lives by making them unable to participate in normal everyday tasks. On top of wanting to avoid these situations, anxiety can make a person feel too weak or fatigued to engage in social activities. This further cements their desire to withdraw and stay confined to their safe space instead of facing and managing their anxiety.

Causes and treatments

Most people feel anxious at some point in their life, but there can be certain factors or triggers that cause other people to feel it more severely than normal. These can include someone's genetics, their environment, how their brain is wired, and what life experiences they've had. If a person associates something with fear, it is likely they will develop anxiety surrounding that thing. Although it is typical for people to have some sort of trigger for their anxiety, this is not true for all cases. Some people have very generalized anxiety about nothing in particular; they are simply always worried or dreading being out in the world.

For some people, one type of anxiety can cause them to develop another type of anxiety. For example, someone who has anxiety about suffering harm or getting sick might develop a germ-related obsessive-compulsive disorder as a way to ensure they will never get sick. Or, people with social anxiety disorder might eventually develop agoraphobia if they never force themselves to interact with others.

Risk factors for different types of anxiety disorders typically coexist in people who suffer with them, which demonstrates that no single experience is likely to cause someone to develop a disorder. Scientists have found that nature and nurture are strongly linked when it comes to the likelihood that someone will develop severe anxiety. Genetically, research has shown that people have about a 30 to 67 percent chance of inheriting anxiety from their parents (Carter, n.d.). Although someone's DNA might be a factor in them developing anxiety, it cannot account for all of the reasons that have developed it.

Environmental factors should also be taken into consideration when trying to find the root cause of anxiety. Parenting style can be a large factor in whether or not a person will develop anxiety. If parents are controlling of their children or if they model anxious behaviors, the child might grow up thinking these are normal behaviors they should model. This can lead to feeling anxious based on a learned behavior. Other factors such as continual stress, abuse, or loss of a loved one can also elicit a severe anxious reaction because a person may not know how to handle the situation they find themselves in.

In addition to the environment, a person's health can often cause anxiety as well. If someone is diagnosed or living with a chronic medical condition or a severe illness, it can cause an anxious reaction. One possibility is if the illness is affecting the person's hormones which can cause stress, or if their feelings of not having control are worsened by a diagnosis they cannot fix.

Some people might not realize that the choices they make daily could be contributing to their anxiety. Things such as excessive caffeine, tobacco use, and not exercising enough can all cause anxiety. Caffeine and other stimulants can increase a person's heart rate and simulate anxiety symptoms. Not exercising can lower a person's level of happy hormones and make their muscles tense or sore which can also contribute to stress. A person's personality can also determine how severe their anxiety might be. Shy people who tend to stay away from conversations and interaction might develop more severe social anxiety because they are not exposed to those situations often.

When experiencing anxiety, it can seem like there is no way out, but there are actually quite a few different ways a person can work to ease their worries, ranging from clinical to holistic approaches. What type of treatments will work depends on the person, and often, how severe their struggle is.

A few clinical ways to treat anxiety include counseling, psychotherapy, and medication. These are not the only ways a person can be medically treated, but they tend to be the most conventional routes for treating mental illness. Counseling is a type of therapy where the person is able to talk to a licensed practitioner and receive feedback and advice about their situation and how to handle their emotions. Most counselors have a master's degree in the psychology field and are licensed through their state. This type of therapy is usually considered a short-term solution for people who are struggling but not debilitated by their anxiety.

Psychotherapy is typically a more long-term solution for people whose lives are impacted by their anxiety. This type of therapy can focus on a broader range of issues and triggers such as a person's anxious patterns or behaviors and how to fix them. Cognitive behavioral therapy is often used in this type of therapy to work with the person to adjust their thoughts and behaviors.

Some people find relief once prescribed medication to help them manage their anxiety. This route is usually reserved for people who are struggling the most and having trouble calming themselves on their own. There are various types of medications such as SSRIs (selective serotonin reuptake inhibitors) and

SNRIs (serotonin-norepinephrine reuptake inhibitors) that alter brain chemicals to reduce anxiety or worry.

Making changes to their lifestyle and habits can also help people with anxiety relieve some of their symptoms. This is a more natural approach to managing anxiety and can be successful for people who are dedicated to making positive life changes. Small things such as diet adjustments and increasing activity levels can reduce anxious feelings. Establishing a consistent sleep schedule is also important to help someone ensure they are getting enough rest each night. Stress fatigues the body and it may need more time to fully recuperate at night if it was taxed during the day. Making sure the body has a routine can also make someone feel safe and know what to expect from their day.

Meditation can also be a good way for people to calm their minds and ease anxiety. Taking time during the day to be still and quiet might help someone stop the constant worry they feel during the day and relax for a moment. Once they start training their body to relax, it is more likely that they can keep it up during the day. Finally, avoiding stimulants such as caffeine, sugar, and tobacco, and depressants such as alcohol can greatly improve a person's chances of overcoming their anxiety. These substances contribute to the brain's hyperactivity and can often increase feelings of anxiety.

Chapter 2: Panic Attacks

Unlike anxiety, not everyone has experienced a panic attack. Panic attacks are the result of extreme levels of anxiety and can sometimes make people feel like they are having a heart attack. Panic attacks typically have similar symptoms to anxiety, but they are experienced in much larger doses and can start suddenly without any particular trigger. If someone has panic attacks frequently enough, they might be diagnosed with panic disorder. Usually a panic attack subsides after no more than half an hour, but these minutes can be long and painful for the person experiencing symptoms.

There are a number of things that can cause a panic attack and what might be the last straw of anxiety before an attack begins depends on the person. It is still unknown what exactly causes panic attacks, but they seem to follow regular anxiety after similar lines and triggers. They can have genetic origins in some families, but life experiences can also contribute to a person's tendency to panic. Other potential causes include medication, whether it is something a person is taking or something they are withdrawing from, and the person's temperament. People who tend to react strongly to situations might be more likely to have panic attacks in stressful situations.

Panic attacks can be incredibly scary, especially in people who experience them frequently. People with panic disorder might benefit from choosing medication to manage their condition at the beginning of treatment because it helps make their symptoms less severe. There are ways to calm oneself down during a panic attack, but it takes practice and time to master the skills. Just like with anxiety, the treatment options are up to the person to decide what might work best for them. This chapter examines what panic attacks are, what it feels like to have one, potential causes, and how they can accumulate into panic disorder.

What is a Panic Attack?

Panic attacks are similar to anxiety, but with much more severe symptoms. A person's racing heart paired with chest pain and dizziness might make their body think they are having a heart attack. Especially for people who have never experienced panic before, realizing that it is an emotional situation and not a physical threat can be the most difficult part of an attack. Some people experience them so often that they qualify as having a panic disorder, which is characterized by having frequent panic attacks that interrupt daily life. They are common in people with heightened anxiety and can be triggered by the same things that spark anxiety.

They are much more than simply feeling worried, though, as they are a full-body response to fear. More specifically, panic attacks are thought to be related to the body's fight or flight response.

When a person feels threatened, their body starts producing adrenaline and readying the muscles to either run or defend itself, while also triggering a fear response. Panic attacks are similar to this reaction but without an imminent threat as a trigger. Sometimes when the body misfires this way, a person can feel like they are in immediate danger, despite not being able to tell what is posing the threat. They might begin associating benign objects or situations with danger because their body panics when confronted with them.

Panic attacks are characterized by their sudden onset and quick peak time, which is usually within a few minutes after the first symptoms appear. There are pros and cons to these qualities; panic attacks typically last only 10-30 minutes, but they can also present severe symptoms out of the blue. The duration and intensity of an attack are what sets it apart from normal anxiety. An anxious person might experience some symptoms for the entire day, but they are mild enough to manage and be able to continue with life. If you're experiencing a panic attack, though, it may only last a few minutes but there is not a way to continue with life during the minutes of panic because the symptoms are too intense.

A panic attack often occurs in tandem with other anxiety disorders and can present when people are in situations that elicit higher levels of anxiety than normal. Often times a person who is attempting to face one of their fears might trigger a panic attack by ignoring their anxiety and causing their brain to increase the fight or flight signals.

Luckily, most people only experience this panic on occasion. The symptoms might make them feel like they are having a heart attack or about to faint, but these are only the physical symptoms of a mental problem. It is important to remember if you are having a panic attack that your body is not in danger and the problem is not physical. People who have panic attacks frequently, such as once a week or every few days, might also notice that their panic attacks last longer than the standard half-hour. When these people seek help, they might be diagnosed with panic disorder. This is similar to anxiety disorders, but instead of free-floating anxiety, the person has panic attacks during the day.

Symptoms of panic attacks can range from a pounding or racing heart to dizziness, nausea, and shortness of breath, among others. To be considered a panic attack and not just severe anxiety, however, a person would have to display at least four symptoms at one time. This helps to distinguish between anxiety and panic attacks because their symptoms are almost identical. The reason some people mistake these symptoms for a heart attack is that they can often feel most severe in someone's chest; heart palpitations, an increased heart rate, chest pain and discomfort, shortness of breath and numbness or tingling are all signs of a panic attack that could be misinterpreted.

Other symptoms a person might experience during a panic attack include excessive sweating, trembling or shaking, and irregular temperature—such as feeling feverish or having chills. These symptoms can happen all at once or in rapid succession, which is what sets them apart from their role in anxiety. People might also feel faint or dizzy during a panic attack and need to sit down, or have stomach pains and feel nauseous. Physical symptoms are not all you might experience, though. Panic attacks often bring on thoughts that you are dying, cause intense fear about something, or make you feel like you are going crazy. This is a unique characteristic of panic attacks: they combine mental stress with physical symptoms that will reinforce negative thoughts. If you think you are in danger of dying, a panic attack's severe symptoms might reinforce the thought that something is wrong with your body or you might die.

Panic attacks can also cause other mental anguish not associated with what started the attack. When someone is having a panic attack, they might suddenly feel embarrassed to be reacting in an abnormal way to a normal situation, or they might feel out of control and like the whole room is wondering what is wrong with them. These hypersensitivities could increase their anxiety and intensify the panic attack even more, contributing to their feelings of terror or danger. This can make someone feel like they have to run away, which can be troublesome in situations where leaving is not an easy option such as in a work meeting or during a class.

When panic symptoms finally subside, a person usually feels worn out or fatigued and might need to rest and recover from the experience. The tired feeling is most likely caused by the adrenaline crash you experience after the attack is over. Even though you may not have been moving, your muscles and body still went through a lot of stress and need time to recover.

Another thing people might experience after a panic attack is the fear of having another one. Just like with any traumatic event, a person will be inclined to avoid anything that could potentially put their body in distress again, even if they aren't sure what triggered the reaction in the first place. This is why people who have frequent panic attacks are also at risk of using avoidance as a coping mechanism. If they think they've figured out what causes their panic attacks, they will likely avoid that situation to try to ensure they will not have another attack.

Causes and Severity

The exact causes of panic attacks are still unknown and hard to pin down because they can vary so much among people. Researchers seem to think the triggers are similar to those of anxiety, and a variety of factors can determine a person's predisposition to having panic attacks. It seems that panic attacks are hereditary; if a person has family members that have panic attacks regularly, they are more likely to have them as well. This suggests genetics might play a role in determining whose anxiety might escalate to an attack.

Other potential triggers include major life events or changes such as moving to a different state or country, getting married, and having a baby. All of these events can mean a drastic change to a person's life and might cause so much anxiety or uncertainty that they panic. They also increase stress levels, which can cause anxiety to spike in a number of different situations such as after the death of a family member, divorce, or being fired from a job. Financial stress can be especially difficult for people to handle and could cause panic attacks if they feel there is no way to remedy the situation.

Medical conditions and physical triggers can also cause panic attacks in some people. A chronic medical condition or terminal diagnosis can trigger an anxious response in people who might immediately worry about the uncertainty their condition presents. The conditions themselves, however, can sometimes be the culprit for anxiety and not necessarily just the person's reaction to them. Some physiological conditions such as mitral valve prolapse, thyroid problems, and low blood sugar can also induce panic attacks by throwing off the balance of hormones in the body. Other physical triggers, such as receiving shots in a doctor's office, might put the body into fight or flight mode because you feel threatened.

What someone puts into their body can also have an effect on their anxiety levels and their risk of a panic attack. Excessive use of stimulants such as recreational drugs and caffeine can put the body into overdrive and increase the likelihood of overreacting to benign stimuli. If a person is taking certain types of medication, such as antidepressants, and attempts to discontinue use too quickly, they can experience panic attacks. This is because these medications often alter brain chemicals and the brain might not be making the chemicals it needs to stay balanced and prevent the fear response.

A person's temperament can also be a factor in whether or not they are more likely to experience panic attacks. If someone typically reacts strongly to situations, whether with anger, sadness, joy, etc. they might also react with intense anxiety to threatening situations where others would not. This intense response is especially likely to result in a panic attack in someone who is already experiencing anxiety.

In extreme circumstances, people might begin having panic attacks due to a change in the way their brain functions. This can be because of an accident that affected the fear center of the brain or other areas that relate to it. It could also be from serious medical conditions that affect the brain and its function. When the brain's function is altered it might be more likely to misfire fear responses and lead to panic attacks.

As mentioned earlier, panic attacks are linked to anxiety, which is why some people refer to panic attacks as anxiety attacks. These two terms refer to the same sudden symptoms and feelings and should not be confused for different afflictions.

Similar to how people can develop an anxiety disorder from long-term anxiety, they can also develop panic disorder if they start having attacks frequently enough. Being diagnosed with a disorder is a sign that your anxiety levels are high enough to be interfering with your life, even if you might not notice it. Panic disorder is usually diagnosed if a person is experiencing attacks at random with no clear trigger for the reaction. Another criterion is that the person must be continually afraid of having another attack, typically to the point of avoiding activities that might bring one on. This disorder typically affects adults, but some children can suffer from it as well. It is more common in adults because they are more prone to continual high-stress situations and have more life experiences that could have possibly cemented a fear in their brain.

Panic disorder affects only about 2 to 3% of people in the United States and most of these people are women. This could be because women are more susceptible to fluctuations in hormones which might contribute to them feeling frequently anxious or worried. The statistic does reflect, though, how rare meeting all of the criteria for panic disorder is.

Just like anxiety, panic disorder can disrupt someone's life by making it impossible for them to leave their homes. They might miss work or school and not be able to turn in assignments on time to save their job or GPA. It can also keep them from performing basic functions such as going to the grocery store for food and leave them dependent on others for care.

Panic disorder also has a variety of treatment options for people who suffer from it. Psychotherapy is one option, where a doctor can assess the situation and help you work through your fears and recognize potential triggers. If the attacks are too difficult to manage on your own, the doctor might suggest medicine to help manage symptoms until you are more confident in your abilities to handle the symptoms of a panic attack.

One way a person might be able to curb the feelings of panic is by practicing mindfulness. A doctor might suggest a few activities or a person can practice mindful tactics on their own. Mindfulness is similar to meditation and focuses on listening to the body and quieting the mind. People who practice mindfulness can learn to ignore their thoughts of stress and worry for an allotted amount of time each day. Once a person learns what it takes for them to reach a peaceful state, they can continue using these activities during the day when they start to feel anxious or overwhelmed.

Chapter 3: Dangers of Anxiety

Living with constant negative thoughts and intense fears can cause someone to wish for a way to ease their pain or to develop unhealthy habits that could make their symptoms worse. Anxiety is linked to a number of other mental illnesses, most notably depression. This combination can cause people to make poor decisions when they are motivated to find relief from their symptoms. Some people will turn to drugs or alcohol, which can make symptoms worse. Other people might find more dangerous ways to cope with their mental problems and cause physical harm to themselves.

Being anxious can also result in people refusing to leave their homes or to only go to certain places that they feel are safe. This can lead to a drastic decrease in social interaction, which can be counterproductive to their healing. Humans are innately social beings and when people take interaction out of their lives, they might experience even more negative thoughts or have trouble noticing when the thoughts are irrational. It can also impede their ability to relate to others socially when they are out of practice and thus further cement their fears that communicating with other people is too painful an activity.

Not all anxiety is likely to pose harm to the person experiencing it. Typically, it takes high levels of constant anxiety to lead a person to attempt to find relief in substances or to completely avoid things they believe cause their anxiety. Once a person starts going down that road, though, it is important to get help as soon as possible. Exposing themselves to the things they are afraid of is often the best way for a person to understand that it is not an actual threat. If people do not have a strong support network to get them through their anxious periods, they may have a harder time getting back to a healthy place.

Negative Effects

One of the hallmark symptoms of anxiety is having a sense of impending doom that you can't shake. This can make it difficult to concentrate during the day or find a moment of peace because there might always be that voice in the back of your head telling you something is wrong. Sometimes this voice can become so loud or be so relentless that it induces a panic attack. The sense of fear and stress that come with panic attacks make it even more difficult to move on with the day after the symptoms have passed.

A sense of doom is not the only negative effect anxiety can have on a person's life, though. As mentioned in the introduction to this chapter, anxiety and depression are often closely linked and it is not uncommon for someone with one of these afflictions to also experience the other, whether it's from time to time or chronic. The combination of these two issues can often cause increased stress in people, which can then lead to headaches or high blood pressure. Sometimes having physical symptoms to match their emotional ones can be too much for a person to handle and might lead to avoidance coping.

The constant discomfort can also contribute to someone becoming irritable or extremely quiet. When you have a headache, it can be difficult to concentrate and having people at school or work demanding that tasks be completed can sometimes cause someone to react angrily because they cannot handle any more stress or focus on projects. On the other hand, some people might become extremely quiet because they prefer to fight their battle on their own or they might think no one would take their struggle seriously if they did voice their pain.

Anxiety can also cause people to believe they are having breathing problems when symptoms start to increase in intensity. When they are distressed their breathing might become shallow and rapid, which makes it hard for the body to get enough oxygen to calm down. Constant anxiety and stress can also contribute to stomach issues in some people. Stress is known to cause stomach ulcers and it is not uncommon for people with anxiety to develop ulcers or other gastrointestinal issues. Some people experience cramping, pain in the abdomen, or develop food sensitivities. Keeping a healthy balanced diet can help anxious people to avoid or alleviate some of these symptoms.

Anxiety can even affect a person's energy levels, especially if they are prone to panic attacks. If the body remains in a constant state of stress, it can wear down the immune system and tire the organs and muscles in the body. This means a person will often need more time to rest so the body can heal itself and have energy for the next day. It also, unfortunately, causes people to have trouble sleeping soundly so they may wear out their body until they do not have enough energy to leave their home. Along with energy, it can also sap someone's libido, which might cause problems in their personal relationships, creating more stress.

Social anxiety disorder is one of the more common anxiety disorders and can seriously affect a person's social life and how they relate to and interact with others. This disorder is characterized by someone experiencing intense anxiety at the thought or act of interacting with others. It can make it difficult for the person to go to parties, speak in front of groups, or even have a conversation. Avoidance strategies as a means of coping is not uncommon in this group. Most people with social anxiety disorder might try to avoid making friends or speaking to others because they are afraid of what the other person might think of them.

Social anxiety goes beyond the normal feelings of nervousness or being shy in public. It is an extreme discomfort that couples with fear to the point that a person might feel they are in danger when they enter a social setting. A person might decide it is not worth it to attempt interacting with others and start withdrawing and keeping to themselves. This can get so severe to the point where the person may be unwilling to attend work or school and might not have a trusted group of friends to discuss their symptoms with.

Common symptoms of social anxiety disorder are constantly worrying about what other people think of you and being overly critical of yourself. These negative interpretations of situations and the self can contribute to someone's fear and worry about interacting with others. They often convince themselves things are going badly before a conversation even starts and then feel embarrassed or humiliated. These fears are paired with the constant worry that someone might notice how anxious they are and call it out in conversation. Anxiety typically causes coping behaviors such as touching the face or twiddling fingers, which a socially anxious person might be hyper-aware of in themselves. These worries often lead to people not interacting with strangers because they are unsure of how they will react.

People with social anxiety also tend to fear being the center of attention, which causes them to go out of their way to stay away from the spotlight. You will rarely see someone with social anxiety auditioning for the lead in a play or offering to speak in front of a group. In situations where they are the center of attention, they might experience symptoms such as sweating, blushing, shaking, or trouble focusing. Once someone begins treating their anxiety, however, these activities might become easier.

When a person with social anxiety does manage to interact with someone else or with a group, they typically spend a considerable amount of time analyzing their mistakes afterward, even if there weren't any. Social anxiety can make someone very critical of themselves which can drive their fears because they believe they are performing at a subpar level when it comes to communicating with others. Expecting the worst-case scenario and then convincing themselves it was the outcome, is how most people with social anxiety typically end up using avoidance to deal with their problems. Once they become convinced their actions only end in failure, they might lose the motivation to continue trying for success.

Panic attacks can also have other negative effects on people besides the terrible symptoms that mark them. They can affect a person's physical and mental health as well as limit their social life by creating a constant circle of being afraid of having an attack. Aside from putting extra stress on the body with increased levels of anxiety, people also tend to pull away socially when they experience panic attacks. They can often lose the people that served as their support group if they begin to withdraw from their friends. Alternately, if you are not willing to explain your symptoms to friends, then they might pull away because they think you do not want to spend time with them.

Losing friends can easily cause someone to socially withdraw even more so they can protect themselves from feeling rejected by others. This can also cement their negative self-criticism that they might not be worth people's time or too awkward for people to want to hang out with them. Even people that you manage to keep in your life despite panic disorder might not be enough to get you through difficult times. People often decrease the frequency they see or speak to their friends if their panic attacks are too much to handle. They might feel too embarrassed to discuss it with a friend or humiliated for not being able to cope on their own.

Panic attacks can also cause financial harm to a person. If they are too anxious to go to work or if working in their office or job triggers panic attacks, a person may stop working for a while or quit altogether. This halt in income can be a stressor for people without anxiety and an easy trigger for people with anxiety. Not being able to attend work increases the likelihood that someone with anxiety or panic attacks might have to claim themselves as disabled. This could be the only way for them to receive income if they are unable to function normally in the workplace.

If panic attacks are frequent enough, a person might also be at an increased risk of suicidal thoughts or tendencies, which can pose a threat to their life. Similar to feelings of hopelessness in those with depression, people who struggle to manage their panic attacks or panic disorder might feel like they do not have any hope of leading a normal life. These feelings can lead to devastating decisions and should always be discussed with a doctor.

People with frequent panic attacks can also develop phobias if they associate a specific thing or situation with their condition. For example, if a person tends to have panic attacks while driving a car, they might associate it with a painful experience and develop a fear of driving.

Some people may not realize that their symptoms are related to anxiety or panic attacks, which could lead them to go to different doctors' offices to find a diagnosis. Typically, any doctor is able to recognize the signs of anxiety, especially in the absence of any other physical problems, and can refer the person to a psychologist. Occasionally, though, a person may not accept that they are struggling mentally and continue to spend money on doctors who cannot help them.

How it Can Harm

Sometimes, people experience more anxiety than they can handle and they turn to self-destructive ways of coping. Persistent anxious feelings can lead to someone physically harming themselves to feel a release from the thoughts that might be suffocating their minds. For some people, it can seem like the only way to manage their symptoms. Anxious feelings such as being overwhelmed or out of control are often triggers for this type of behavior. Some people self-harm because they might feel it gives them some control over their pain when they feel they have lost control over their mind.

There are two types of anxiety that are considered more likely to lead to self-harm: social anxiety and generalized anxiety. People with social anxiety might use self-harm as a way to punish themselves for being inadequate. People with generalized anxiety are usually more likely to use self-harm as a way to relieve the stress and worry they constantly feel. Although obsessive-compulsive disorder is no longer considered an anxiety disorder, people who are diagnosed with it often experience a considerable amount of anxiety surrounding their obsession. This anxiety can lead to self-harm in people with OCD, as well as a way for them to feel in control.

For people with anxiety, self-harm can be a way to momentarily quiet the worried and negative thoughts in their minds. They can often feel that harming themselves provides an outlet for the negativity and a type of release from the pain for themselves. In other, typically more severe cases, a person will have suffered from anxiety for so long that they might feel they are numb to normal emotions. Causing physical pain to themselves can be a way of regaining feelings they might feel they have lost due to the prolonged struggle with anxiety.

Perhaps the most destructive type of self-harm is those who do it out of anger. Some people, usually those with social anxiety, will use self-harm out of anger toward themselves. If they feel they were not good enough or did not try hard enough they might harm themselves as a form of punishment. They might also feel they need to be punished if they are struggling with managing their symptoms on their own. This type of self-harm can be the most dangerous because it is usually a sign of a deeper emotional issue that a person needs to address.

A 2014 study published in the Journal of the Royal Society of Medicine looked at which people were more likely to harm themselves due to a chronic illness. The researchers found that people with chronic mental illness were significantly more likely to self-harm than people with chronic physical illnesses (Goldacre, 2014).

Common risk factors for people who use self-harm as a coping mechanism include depression, anxiety, and alcohol abuse. This could be because these three things can all alter the way a person thinks and the decisions they make. If you find yourself wanting to use self-harm as a coping mechanism, or you are using it, you should seek medical attention as soon as possible. There are many healthy ways to cope with anxiety and panic attacks and a qualified professional can help you find an appropriate outlet.

Chapter 4: Why Anxiety Happens

The causes of panic attacks vary greatly and depend on the person experiencing anxiety. Things such as genetics, the environment, activity level, and diet can all affect someone's level of anxiety. Perhaps the most common cause of anxiety is past experiences because that is typically how people learn to react to situations. If someone had a series of particularly bad experiences at baseball games, they might develop anxiety in baseball stadiums or when asked to play the sport (depending on what the negative experience was). These connections between negative feelings and normal events can cause either anxiety someone outgrows or anxiety that sticks with them.

Although past experiences are the most common trigger for anxiety, genetics cannot be ignored. Scientists have been researching the link between genes and anxiety for years and are making considerable headway in the field. Multiple studies have found links between certain genes and their variations, and anxiety. Some of these genes are inherited from family members and others' expressions can be determined by the person's body and brain. Studies have been done on brain chemicals and their effects on anxiety as well as on twins to study gene expression and find correlations to other family members.

Environmental factors, both past and present, can also determine a person's level and type of anxiety. If a person grew up in an environment where anxious behavior was presented as the norm, they might have trouble breaking anxious habits as an adult. In today's world, social media can also cause a considerable amount of anxiety in people who are unable to unplug from it. They might constantly feel like they have not obtained the social approval they need to be fulfilled and develop social anxiety from constant self-doubt. This chapter will broadly explore potential causes and triggers for anxiety and panic attacks including genetics, environmental factors, and past experiences.

Causes

People all experience anxiety differently, which means they are all triggered by different things. The source of each person's anxiety varies based on their life experiences, genetics, and environment. A person typically develops fear from a negative experience or series of experiences, that caused their brain to associate danger or pain with an object or situation. It can also appear in adulthood due to a major life change that makes a person feel uncertain about their future. For example, if someone is diagnosed with terminal cancer, they will most likely feel anxious about their suddenly shortened future. This anxiety turns into a problem, however, when it becomes all-consuming and the person is unable to move on from their initial feelings.

In addition to medical diagnosis, medication can also cause anxiety in some people. Some prescription medicines, such as birth control pills, can adjust a person's hormone levels and sometimes result in an imbalance. Other medications such as cold medicines and certain weight loss pills have potent active ingredients that could make someone feel on edge and possibly trigger anxiety if the symptoms are close enough. Substances can also trigger anxiety and sometimes panic attacks. The biggest culprit here is caffeine. Caffeine can be a powerful stimulant for some people, which means it might put their bodies on high alert if they consume too much. Once on high alert, their body might signal the alarm to things that are not a threat because it is on edge and already producing adrenaline.

Even simple things such as skipping meals can contribute to anxiety. This is because when a person does not eat, they often experience a blood sugar crash or low blood sugar, which can mimic symptoms of anxiety or a panic attack with shaky hands or dizziness. When people feel these symptoms, they might assume they are feeling anxious and then become more anxious if they do not know what brought on the initial feelings.

Financial concerns are another common cause of anxiety. Saving money or being in debt can be incredibly stressful for some people and might result in constant anxiety about their financial situation. Luckily, this anxiety can be easily reduced by visiting a financial advisor and establishing a savings plan.

Possibly the most common cause of anxiety, both in people with and without anxiety, is parties and social events. Most people feel uncomfortable when first arriving at an event involving many people because they might not know who to talk to or what to say. If you have social anxiety, however, this setting can be especially uncomfortable. You might spend the whole night feeling inadequate and wondering if people are judging you. Public events such as festivals or having to speak in front of a group of people are other common triggers for social anxiety.

A final common cause of anxiety is conflict. Fighting with a loved one or spouse can be stressful for anyone, but for people who struggle with anxiety, it can be especially scary. The person might feel like the argument is their fault or that they will lose the relationship because they have upset the other person. Navigating conflict with anxiety is difficult because a person often does not have an accurate view of what is happening due to their self-criticism.

Sometimes the fuel behind the fire is not as common as the causes listed above. Genetic factors can also determine whether or not a person will develop anxiety and possibly even the severity of their anxiety. A genetic link paired with environmental factors can sometimes be the perfect cocktail of anxiety for someone. Some researchers have even found links and correlations between specific genes and chromosomes and genetic anxiety. In some cases, the condition was inherited from one of their parents and in others, it is simply how the gene expresses itself that causes anxiety.

A 2002 study showed that the specific expression of a serotonin transporter gene can be correlated with a person's type of anxiety (Morris-Rosendahl, 2002). This means that the way that particular gene interacts with their body could mean the difference between someone developing social anxiety or generalized anxiety. Another study in 2015 looked at newborn twins and found that a specific gene variation can increase a person's risk of developing generalized anxiety disorder (Burri, 2015). These two studies show how gene expression can play a huge role in whether or not someone will develop anxiety.

In 2016, researchers examined how genetics could cause generalized, social, and panic disorder. They found that certain genes interact with hormones and other things in the body in a certain way that increased a person's risk of developing these disorders (Domschke, 2016). Finally, a 2017 study showed that generalized anxiety disorder is, in fact, inheritable. The scientists performed research on both families and twins to study the links between a variety of genes that cause generalized anxiety disorder and saw that those were being passed down to children.

Genetic risk for developing anxiety can be a complicated web, though. Although scientists have identified some specific genes that contribute to certain disorders, it can still be a combination of which genes a person receives and how they are expressed that can determine that person's anxiety level.

It can sometimes be difficult for a person to tell if anxiety runs in their family, however, mostly because anxiety can present itself a number of ways and is different in each person. Also, if the person comes from a more reserved family, their family member may never mention that they manage anxiety daily. Typically, anxiety due to genetics begins at a young age. Most people who experience anxiety because of genetic factors first start noticing symptoms before they are 20 years old. This can be a sure sign that anxiety runs in the family, especially if there are few other risk factors in the person's life.

Genetic factors can, however, go hand-in-hand with environmental factors for some people. These causes can be based on a person's personal experiences or determined by the environment they live or work in. Despite the personalization of these causes, there are some common triggers that might affect people.

Stress is probably the most common environmental factor that is central to a person's anxiety. Stress often causes people to worry excessively and can cause or exacerbate anxiety. It can be both a cause and a side effect of the negative thoughts and feelings someone experiences when they are anxious.

Trauma is another common cause of anxiety in people who have had profoundly negative experiences. Trauma at any age can cause lasting anxiety, but most people with persistent anxiety have experienced a traumatic event as a child. Going through something difficult at a young age can greatly increase a person's risk of developing an anxiety disorder. Life events that lack a positive ending can also cause a person to develop anxiety surrounding similar situations. Things such as the baseball game example given earlier can affect them throughout their entire life if they do not make efforts to alleviate that fear.

The way a person was raised can also have a major impact on whether or not they will develop anxiety as an adult. Particularly for people who were raised by anxious parents, it can be difficult to discern normal behaviors from anxious ones once they are grown up. This is because a child learns behaviors from their parents and if they are exhibiting anxious behaviors that will become the child's norm, they might even develop anxious behaviors before anxiety, but the two go hand-in-hand regardless.

Social media can also contribute to a person's anxiety. Excessive use of social media can even lead to depression if a person is unable to unplug and interact with others in real life. Social interactions over the web are based on positive feedback and if a person does not receive what they believe is an appropriate amount it can lead to self-doubt and negative self-talk which can create anxiety when they are around others. The increased use of social media has also given people unlimited access to news stories and information from across the world. This can create a sense that the world is a much more dangerous place than it is because you are constantly exposed to negative stories. Sometimes this is enough to cause anxiety in people who might feel they will be harmed if they leave their homes or interact with a stranger.

Relationships can be another cause of anxiety for some people, especially those who struggle socially. They might have feelings related to not being good enough for their partner or cannot connect the way they need to. A relationship can also cause anxiety if the person is ready to end it but afraid to cause a conflict by breaking up with their partner.

Cultural differences are a seldom considered social factor that can make people feel anxious in social situations as well. For someone who has just moved to a new country, it might be intimidating to interact with native people because they are not aware of all the rules or customs. You might be afraid of saying the wrong thing and embarrassing either yourself or someone else.

Who is at Risk?

With all of these risk factors, you might be wondering if there is a group of people who are more likely to develop anxiety. Although there are some correlations between certain groups, anxiety is actually the most common mental illness in the United States. It affects about 40 million adults in the country, about

18% of people (ADAA, n.d.). Anxiety and the disorders that come with it can be easily treated by doctors, but many people choose not to seek help. This is perhaps one of the reasons anxiety is one of the most widespread mental issues.

Statistically, people who suffer from depression are more likely to also suffer from anxiety. This could be because the two conditions occur in the same part of the brain but affect people differently. It could also be because when people are overly critical of themselves, they might become convinced they are not good enough for others and feel depressed. Studies also show that women are twice as likely to develop generalized anxiety or panic disorder than men. This could be contributed to higher levels of certain hormones that could affect the brain and stress responses. It could also be due to high levels of stress in the increasing number of women who work and raise children.

Social anxiety seems to affect men and women almost equally, but typically has an earlier onset than other types of anxiety. People often start noticing their first symptoms of social anxiety when they are about 13 years old. From their first symptoms, the majority of people wait at least a decade before seeking help.

Often times, people with other illnesses, whether mental or physical, will be more likely to develop anxiety than a healthy person. This could be contributed to the increased stress that person feels in dealing with their illness daily, or the stress their body is put through while trying to fight off the illness. A few particular ailments have been linked to anxiety, including cardiovascular disease, COPD (chronic obstructive pulmonary disease), diabetes, and cancer. All of these diagnoses can be long-term illnesses and come with a host of their own complications that might have a person on a slew of medications or visiting the doctor's office often.

The region a person lives in can even have an impact on whether or not they will experience anxiety. For example, people living in North America are more likely to have anxiety than anywhere else in the world. This could be contributed to the fast-paced, work-focused lifestyle in the U.S. and parts of Canada, developing higher levels of stress among people.

Age can also be a factor in who is most likely to experience anxiety. Typically, if children will have anxiety it will be between the ages of 13 and 18. In adults, people under 35 years old are the most likely to feel anxious, possibly because of financial stress that older adults do not experience as intensely.

Chapter 5: Anxious Behavior

People might think that anxiety is only an internal struggle, but there are actually quite a few signals a person might display when they are anxious. Anxiety does not stay just in someone's mind; worried thoughts can often make a person act a certain way as a way to avoid feeling any more anxiety than they have to. Some behaviors are readily apparent, such as tapping their fingers on a desk or touching their face often, and others are not as easy to spot, such as when a person starts withdrawing or isolating themselves. Both can be noticed, though, if a person knows what to look for.

Anxious behavior is usually a way for the person to cope with their feelings through outward expression. For example, if a person is feeling anxious in a meeting, they might think they feelings will subside if they leave, so they may start rapidly bouncing their leg as a way to feel like they are moving and not stuck in an uncomfortable situation. Other ways of coping are not healthy for people, such as when they turn to stimulants or depressants to mask their symptoms. It can be easy for an anxious person to choose something that alleviates their symptoms immediately, but this can make symptoms worse if they aren't dealing with the underlying issue.

There are ways a person can become aware of their own anxious behaviors such as being mindful or keeping a journal. There are also coping mechanisms they can use to calm themselves down enough to be able to rationally think through their fears or worries. This chapter discusses different anxious behaviors, why people might display these behaviors, ways to become aware of them, and methods to cope with the anxiety that causes them.

What Does It Look Like?

Everyone has seen a nervous person before. Sometimes they are easy to spot and other times it is more difficult, but a person can always notice their demeanor by watching their behavior. When people feel anxious they usually show signs in the way they sit, what they do with their hands, and where they are looking.

The first thing you might notice if someone is anxious is that they will seem restless or agitated. Anxious people sometimes have trouble sitting still, so they tend to shake their leg or tap their fingers in an attempt to occupy their mind. This activity can also demonstrate that they are ready to leave the situation because it is making them too anxious. Alternatively, some people might become more and more still and start to withdraw from others socially. This can be because their fear of interacting becomes too much for them to ignore. If friends are not mindful of someone's behavior, they may not notice that the person is suffering from anxiety and think they are simply pulling away from the group. A common trigger for people who react this way is crowds, so they might start avoiding parties and festivals and stay home instead.

Just like some people with anxiety might withdraw from social situations, others may avoid them entirely. If a person's anxiety is severe enough, they might limit the activities they do in a day to only those that do not cause symptoms in an effort to reduce their anxiety during the day.

Another way you might be able to tell if someone is anxious is by their level of organization. Sometimes people who are anxious have trouble focusing and therefore might have trouble organizing their thoughts and tasks. This can mean falling behind at work, or not being able to keep up with their home. Feeling like you can't keep your head above water at work and in your personal life can be incredibly frustrating. For someone with anxiety, it might cause them to feel angry and irritable and react negatively to other people in their life as a way to deal with their own frustration.

People who are anxious are often startled easily because their body is already on edge. They could also be jumpy because their brain has put their body on high alert and is ready to defend itself. If you notice someone who seems particularly jumpy or on edge, ask them if everything is okay so they have the opportunity to talk through their feelings if they would like to.

Other people might become attached to an object or place that makes them feel safe. This could be a watch or necklace that the person believes keeps their anxiety at bay or any other object that makes them feel safe. As far as places, most people feel safest in their home and choose to stay there if they experience anxiety in public. The problem with this behavior is that it can often worsen symptoms. When a person listens to their anxiety and does not confront their fears, they reinforce that fear and possibly make their anxiety worse when they eventually do have to face it.

How to Handle Anxious Behavior

Behavior changes are common in most anxiety disorders and might be the first sign that a friend or family member is struggling. Knowing the signs can help you to step in before symptoms get too severe and start interfering with the person's life. Perhaps the most common sign to look for is moping around and withdrawing from others. Someone with anxiety often feels sad, frustrated, and fatigued from worry. It can seem natural to them to take a step back and keep to themselves to recharge. This can have adverse effects on their mental health, however, and should be addressed if someone notices it. People need social stimulation to maintain a healthy image of themselves and to receive things such as approval and acceptance. If someone begins to limit their exposure to other people, they can miss out on these important things and get trapped in their own self-critical thoughts.

Some people with panic disorder might also withdraw, but for different reasons. These people often associate places with panic attacks so they might avoid an area or situation that they believe will cause a panic attack. For example, if someone had a particularly intense panic attack at the mall one day, they might begin to avoid the mall because they think going inside will cause them to have another panic attack. These situations can get severe enough that the person refuses to leave their home because they feel it is the only safe space for them.

Compulsive behaviors can also be a signal of anxiety. Some people use certain behaviors to curb their anxiety and if they help enough, it might become compulsive. For example, some people will turn the lights on and off a certain number of times before leaving the house to ease their worry that the lights are not off when they leave the house. Some compulsive behaviors, especially in people with OCD, can be directly linked to a specific phobia or fear. This is demonstrated, for instance, in people who might be afraid of germs so they obsessively clean their homes to ensure they are not in danger of getting sick.

Nervous tics can also develop if someone experiences anxiety for a prolonged amount of time. These can range from a restless leg to touching the face, winking or blinking excessively, or even taking a sip of a beverage when an anxious thought pops into your mind. Similar to nervous tics are bad habits that a person develops as a way to cope with their anxiety. These are different from tics because a person is more aware of them and could potentially break the habit if they focus hard enough.

Unfortunately, not all anxious behaviors are as benign as seeming sad or repeating an activity. Some people turn to drugs or alcohol to help mask the pain associated with their anxiety or to quiet their anxious thoughts during the day. This coping mechanism can also lead to worsening symptoms because it masks the problem instead of addressing it.

If someone wanted to change or address their anxious behaviors, they would need to start being mindful of their actions and decisions. This means they would need to acknowledge when they perform the behavior and then try to figure out what might be causing it. If they can find the core of the problem it can be much easier to solve. The easiest way to do this is to ask "why" after a negative behavior. This allows the person to find their motivation and determine if it is negative or positive and what effect the decision might have on their mental health.

Once a person accomplishes mindfulness, they should employ a strong support system of friends and family to help them stick with their plan to eliminate anxious behaviors. These people can help you stay on track and might even have insight as to what is causing your anxiety. It can also give you someone to turn to on days you feel overwhelmed. It can be difficult to know what to do next when dealing with anxiety, but having a network of people to support and guide you can offer much-needed help and clarity in difficult situations.

Another way to treat anxious behavior is to treat the anxious thoughts as the root cause. If a person focuses on eliminating the thoughts that lead to the behavior, they can usually manage to reduce or stop the behavior altogether. They will usually need to use certain tactics to calm their anxious thoughts before they cause negative behavior for this method to succeed. The key focus in this exercise should be determining if the fear a person feels is warranted or not. They should consider their anxious thoughts and then analyze the situation to see if there is a real threat or if it is just their fear making them anxious. If they can manage to see that their fear is driving most of their anxious thoughts, a person may be able to find some relief from their anxious behaviors. Seeing that their fear is not rational or based on anything concrete can often be helpful in alleviating anxiety itself also.

People can also make sure they are educated about their type of anxiety to make themselves more aware of its effects and associated behaviors. If someone knows what they are looking for in themselves, it can be much easier to find causes and triggers. Another way to increase self-awareness is to start keeping a journal. Writing down your thoughts and feelings consistently can help you notice patterns and common denominators in your anxiety. It can be difficult to piece together similarities in the moment, but having a written record to go back over can make the process easier.

Finding the best way to track anxiety can take some trial and error and is not always a seamless process. Some people might have to try a few different strategies before they find something that works with their schedule, abilities, and anxiety type. It is important to push forward even if finding the cause of anxiety seems difficult or unfruitful, and not to be afraid to switch methods if what you're doing doesn't seem to be working.

Aside from learning to recognize anxious behavior, most people also want to learn how to cope with their anxiety. Learning how to calm down can be the most difficult yet beneficial thing a person with anxiety can teach themselves. They can use mindfulness techniques such as focusing on only one thing and engaging all of their senses to take their mind away from anxiety.

Exercise can also be an effective way to relieve anxiety. It allows the body to work through the adrenaline it has created and return to a more relaxed state, as well as release hormones that promote happiness. Exercising can be helpful to loosen muscles and promote healthy blood flow, which can both be affected by anxiety.

After exercising, or during a slow or stressful point in the day, a person can also use relaxation exercises to help calm their anxiety. When people find a method that helps them to calm down, even at anxious points during the day, they can have a greater likelihood of managing their anxiety. There are a couple of techniques a person can use to calm down, one of them being muscle relaxation exercises. A person can focus on one muscle at a time and tense that muscle for about 30 seconds, then release the muscle for about 30 seconds. When they release the muscle, they should focus on that feeling of letting go and let it apply to their mind. Deep breathing can also be helpful because it promotes calmness. Anxiety often causes a person to take quick, shallow breaths which can sometimes make the brain feel like it is not getting enough air. When you take a deep breath, your body is able to take in more oxygen and distribute that in your body, relaxing the muscles and mind.

Meditation is another way people can practice calming their anxiety. Most meditative practices are exercises in mindfulness and revolve around being capable of clearing the mind. People with anxiety sometimes find relief in these activities because they give their brain something peaceful to focus on instead of the anxious thoughts buzzing around in their heads.

Limiting caffeine intake can also help some people reduce their anxiety. As discussed earlier, caffeine is a stimulant that can often contribute to increased levels of anxiety, especially if someone experiences symptoms regularly. Avoiding alcohol can also be a good idea if you want to reduce your anxiety. Alcohol is a depressant, and although it may temporarily relieve symptoms, it usually makes them worse in the long-term. This is both because of how it affects the brain and because people who drink alcohol as a coping mechanism are not addressing the root of their problem.

A balanced, healthy diet can help some people reduce their anxiety by reducing the likelihood of experiencing gastrointestinal issues. This can be particularly helpful for people whose anxiety is connected to a stomach issue such as irritable bowel syndrome or Crohn's disease. Keeping a diet that won't irritate the gut can help you be less worried about symptoms flaring up when you are away from your home.

If you are suffering from anxiety and your symptoms are too intense to manage on your own, a doctor can also assist you by prescribing a medication to lessen the symptoms so you can learn how to cope with your anxiety. It is important to remember that not everyone is capable of managing their anxiety alone and it is okay to ask for help.

Chapter 6: Panic Attack Warning Signs

Panic attacks tend to be like bombs of compounded anxiety, constantly ticking with no countdown timer. The suddenness and seeming unpredictability can put people who are already anxious even more on edge. There are some warning signs that indicate a panic attack may be moments away, though, if people know what to look for. They often mimic symptoms of anxiety but can be much more intense and come on just as unexpectedly as panic attacks. Things such as chest pain, racing heart, sweating, and shortness of breath, if presented more intensely than with normal anxiety, can be signs that someone is nearing panic territory.

These responses are not all mental, however. Even though panic attacks are linked to anxiety, a mental illness, the body does have physiological responses to the feelings of dread and worry that cause them. Certain parts of the nervous system start activating parts of the body so it is ready for a fight or flight response, and even the brain activates particular centers that have to do with fear responses and pain experiences. Combined with increased heart rate and blood sugar, a person can feel wired physically while their mind races through its own anxiety.

Luckily, there are ways a person can calm down once a panic attack has started and even decrease the likelihood of experiencing them altogether. Practicing techniques such as deep breathing, muscle relaxation, and mindfulness can help people stop their minds from spiraling out of control and bring their focus back to the present. If a person wants to stop panic attacks from happening, they need to be aware of the signs and be ready with calming techniques to quell the symptoms before they start in earnest. This chapter discusses signs and symptoms of panic attacks, different techniques for calming down once a panic attack starts, and ways to be diligent enough to keep them from happening.

Signs and Symptoms

Despite their sudden onset, there can be signs that a panic attack is about to start. The signs are usually the same symptoms that occur during a panic attack, but they will be less severe for a few minutes before the panic attack starts. This can also depend on the person and how they experience panic attacks or if they have particular triggers.

While experience anxiety, you might notice your heart rate speed up or your heart start beating harder and harder until it is pounding in your chest. These can be precursors to a panic attack while your brain kicks the fight or flight response into high gear and begins to flood your system with adrenaline. In addition to your heart rhythms shifting, you might also notice yourself getting dizzy or lightheaded. It can be tempting to attribute these symptoms to the pounding heart and determine you are having some type of cardiac episode, but it is most likely anxiety turning into panic.

Sometimes even someone's train of thought can be a sign of an impending panic attack. Anxiety often causes thoughts of worry, but a person who is about to have a panic attack might find themselves suddenly fixated on the idea that they are about to die or that are no longer in control of themselves.

Other physical symptoms that can warn someone of a panic attack include sweating, trembling, and shortness of breath. They might feel like they are in the middle of running a marathon while sitting down because the body is convinced that's what it will have to do soon. Nausea and stomach pain can be indicative of panic before the attack begins, as well. The body might be under so much stress it has trouble processing the hormones and chemicals that are flooding its systems, which can result in these two gastrointestinal symptoms.

Temperature regulation is another thing people might start having trouble with before a panic attack sets in. They might become suddenly hot or get chills as the body switches from calm to panic mode. This could be because of the blood rushing to or from muscles as the body prepares itself to fight or run. Some people might notice these symptoms along with the sudden urge to cry or difficulty breathing. Their throat and chest might tighten as they feel their eyes fill with tears; it can seem unwarranted for a minute or two before the panic starts.

A seemingly less intense warning sign that a panic attack is on its way is the feeling of detachment or depersonalization. A person might suddenly feel like they are in a dream or movie and have trouble adjusting their brain to realize it is real life. Or with depersonalization, they might feel like they are watching themselves through a window or from far away. These two symptoms can be serious signs of underlying disorders and should never be ignored.

All of these signs and symptoms can be indicative of both anxiety and panic attacks, but the severity is what you want to watch out for. More severe symptoms can usually tell you a panic attack is on its way and not just your regular bout of anxiety.

Panic attacks might be best known for their physical symptoms and side effects, but there are also a number of physiological components to them as well. People often chalk them up to an emotional reaction to something, but the body physically reacts to the emotions in a lot of interesting ways.

When a person is stressed, the sympathetic nervous system (part of the autonomic nervous system) turns on and starts pumping adrenaline and preparing muscles for the fight or flight response. It responds to various triggers from the brain, such as fear or anxiety, to tell it when to flip the switch. This system, however, has a partner that is supposed to counteract it and keep the balance: the parasympathetic nervous system. This system is in charge of calming down the body, but in some cases, it is not able to do its job in time to keep someone from feeling anxious.

If a person's parasympathetic system cannot calm down their body and stop the flow of adrenaline, then the person will remain on edge and the sympathetic system will stay in control. This means the fight or flight feeling will continue building until the person acts on it and feels they have eliminated the threat. Sometimes, though, a person might not be able to identify what is causing them anxiety or it may not be a physical object, so they cannot remove it from their surroundings. In these situations, the adrenaline can keep flowing, causing anxiety to build up until it turns into a panic attack.

Another part of the fight or flight response is an increase in heart rate so that blood is distributed quickly to the muscles in case they are needed to act on a moment's notice. This increase can cause the cardiac symptoms people typically feel when having anxiety or a panic attack. Breathing often becomes quick and shallow as well in the body's attempt to take in more oxygen and stay on high alert. As discussed with deep breathing, however, this can actually be counterintuitive for people who are trying to calm their bodies down and slow down their minds.

A person's blood sugar also tends to spike during a panic attack with everything else. What goes up must come down though, which means most people experience a blood sugar crash after a panic attack. This is often the cause of post-attack fatigue and lightheadedness.

Scientists have also studied the brain during anxiety and panic attacks and found some interesting information. They have noticed that some parts of the brain become more active than others during a panic attack, such as the amygdala, which is also referred to as the "fear center" of the brain. Certain parts of the midbrain also light up when someone is in a panic. These parts of the brain are responsible for a multitude of functions, including people's pain experience and their defense mechanisms. Finding activity in these two areas of the brain could explain why people feel intense fear during panic attacks and why the body turns on its defense response as a reaction.

Calming Down

When a panic attack starts it might feel like it is never going to end. There are ways, however, that a person can calm themselves down during a panic attack. Most of the tactics to do this consist of taking a moment to breathe, focus, and think clearly. Sometimes the simplest way to ease feelings of panic is to simply acknowledge the feelings and remind yourself they are only temporary. Sometimes this act alone can be enough for a person to relax so they can rationally think through their emotions.

Focusing on breathing can also help relieve some symptoms of a panic attack, similar to how it counteracts anxiety. A person can focus on taking long, deep breaths both as a way to calm their body and to focus their mind on something other than the panic. This can be helpful because when some people start to feel their thoughts spiraling out of control, they might be tempted to follow that negative path deeper into a forest of anxiety. Deep breathing can help you take a moment to realize where your thoughts are leading you and stop following them before you end up deeper in panic.

Another, perhaps more difficult tactic to calm a panic attack is to force yourself to think positively. When negative thoughts start to take over the mind it might be easier to give into them, but fighting them can sometimes keep a person calm. Even if they have to say positive things in an anxious voice, focusing on good messages can help to keep anxiety at a minimum.

Some people might experience most of their panic attacks in social situations when they are trying to adhere to social norms that might be difficult for them. If social conventions are the source of anxiety, then people should not feel pressured to follow them. For example, someone sitting at a dinner table with friends might need to excuse themselves in the middle of the meal to calm down. Worrying about whether or not it is appropriate to leave the table could even cause more stress that would add to the anxiety. They should remember that taking care of themselves is their top priority and not pleasing others.

Mindfulness can help with panic attacks just as it helps with anxiety. People who feel they are starting to panic or who might be afraid their symptoms are not subsiding can try to focus on one thing at a time to get their mind off of the negative thoughts. Sometimes during a panic attack, a person might need something more engaging than staring at an object, so games like Solitaire or Sudoku might be a good way to focus their mind entirely on something else.

If the panic attack is due to overstimulation, however, a person can try closing their eyes or ears to stop their exposure to stimuli and reduce the stress associated with it. To try to avoid other occurrences of this type of panic attack, a person can make sure to be aware of their surroundings. If they notice they are entering a situation with a lot of noise or light, they can begin calming exercises before their anxiety gets a head start on the symptoms and possibly avoid a panic attack.

Some people get good enough at calming themselves down from panic attacks and are able to end them quicker than if they ran their own course. Others, though, want to find a way to stop their panic attacks altogether. The most effective way to do this is to find ways to manage the underlying issue: anxiety. If a person can start to notice the signs of a panic attack, they are also noticing signs of increased anxiety. The trick is to start identifying these symptoms before they become so intense that they are the only thing a person can focus on.

One way to accomplish this is to confront the fears that induce panic attacks. Most people avoid things that induce their panic attacks, but as mentioned earlier, this can actually make symptoms more intense. If they can gradually expose themselves to what they are afraid of, they can become accustomed to it and experience less severe anxiety in relation to it.

Keeping in touch with yourself is another effective way to limit the frequency of panic attacks. Anxiety is different for every person who experiences it, so knowing your personal type of anxiety and what symptoms come with it can be the easiest way to acknowledge when you might be on the edge of panic. This can also help a person recognize when they are starting to feel overwhelmed so they can take a step back and assess what is causing that feeling. Some people either don't notice the feeling right away or try to ignore it, which can lead to further build-up of anxiety over time and eventually a panic attack.

Developing a greater focus can also be effective for people to relieve some anxiety and possibly prevent panic attacks. When they notice their symptoms starting to flare up, picking one object to observe in detail can help focus the mind elsewhere until the symptoms pass. People can also think of the "HALT" method, which stands for hungry, angry, lonely, tired. These are four common triggers for anxiety and panic attacks that people typically do not consider when they realize they are feeling anxious or agitated. If you can focus on yourself and what your body needs, you might be able to realize your anxiety is simply due to one of these four common, and easy to fix causes. Anxious thoughts can often lead a person down a path of "what-ifs." Learning to focus on the present instead of on all the hypotheticals your brain can create can help someone keep their composure in the face of anxiety.

If someone feels their fear building up and threatening a panic attack, they can even do something as simple as grabbing a piece of paper and writing down a rating of intensity of their fear from 1 to 10. This gives them a visual representation of their emotions that might help reduce the sense that it is all in their head. They can continue rating their symptoms every few minutes and watch as the intensity decreases back to a normal level.

Chapter 7: Dealing with Anxiety

Environment can have a large impact on whether or not someone will experience anxiety or a panic attack. Depending on the person's type of anxiety, any range of environments could threaten an attack. Knowing how to deal with these possibilities, though, is key to facing fears and keeping life moving at a normal pace. There are a number of techniques a person can use to manage their anxiety on a daily basis so they don't have to combat it only when it flares up and feels unmanageable. These include mindfulness, eating healthy, exercising, and getting enough sleep each night.

Panic attacks and anxiety can even threaten people in public, sometimes making it especially difficult to deal with because they might feel embarrassed or afraid. Finding ways to ride out the waves of anxiety instead of trying to force them down to deal with later, can be the most helpful way to manage these feelings when a person is a group or out in public. This chapter lists some environments that might make people feel anxious, as well as how to prepare oneself to remain calm in them, how to stave off panic in public, and how to know when it's time to call it quits and head home.

Anxious Environments

The environment a person is in is also a factor in anxiety. Depending on their particular fears, a wide range of situations could cause someone to feel unsafe or afraid and trigger an anxious reaction. The situations that trigger anxiety are typically related to the type of anxiety someone has, such as social or generalized. People with generalized anxiety might have a more difficult time discerning their triggering environments because their anxiety may not be connected to any one situation. Sometimes for these people, the level of tension in a room can be enough of an environmental factor to cause anxiety. Other times they might be nervous that their environment does not have the amenities they need. For example, if someone's anxiety revolves around being afraid they cannot find a bathroom in the event of becoming physically ill, they might have anxiety in a new place where the bathroom is not readily apparent or available.

People with social anxiety tend to dread environments where interacting with others is inevitable. Situations like parties, clubs, and business meetings might all be places where they would feel on edge and more likely to experience anxiety. Typically, their anxiety stems from a fear that others will judge them for how they act or speak, and think they are strange for being different. This can be the motivation behind avoiding situations such as speaking in public or meeting new people. It is important for people with social anxiety to remember, however, that interacting with others is the only way to overcome their fears and start to feel comfortable in groups.

With panic disorder, reactions to the environment might be stronger than simply feeling anxious. Certain environments that are overly stimulating or cause anxiety can often lead a person to have panic attacks. For this reason, this group of people can sometimes be more likely to avoid these triggering environments. Typically, this is a behavior in people with more severe symptoms because they feel they have a greater chance of panicking in public. If you are afraid of leaving your home or don't feel safe in other places, sleeping over at a friend's house might be a triggering environment for you. This can prove especially true if a person has had a panic attack while attempting to attend a sleepover in the past.

Phobias can also be affected by the environment a person is in, especially if that phobia is an object. For example, if someone is afraid of lamps, they might have an incredibly difficult time walking through a home furnishing store or sitting in someone's living room. In a more common example, someone with agoraphobia would experience intense fear or discomfort if they were forced to leave their house. In this scenario, almost any environment that isn't their home could trigger their anxiety.

Although anxious environments can vary from person to person, it is important to remember that avoidance is not the answer. If a certain situation is difficult for you or you believe it will elicit anxiety or a panic attack, then start to ease yourself into it until you begin feeling more comfortable. This can not only help you face your fear but also help your brain release the anxiety by showing it there is no threat.

If a person can recognize what environments cause them anxiety, it can suddenly become much easier to deal with those feelings. The trick to managing symptoms, however, is to catch them before they start and find ways to keep your body calm and in control.

One way to accomplish this is for a person to take time during the day to be quiet and mindful. They can achieve this by doing activities, such as yoga or meditation, that focus on clearing the mind and focusing on the body. These practices give you a chance to quiet your mind and set a positive tone that can persist throughout your day.

Another trick to keeping the mind and body balanced is to maintain an eating schedule so you are never depleted of energy or nutrients. This can also help to stave off the blood sugar crash that comes with hunger mentioned earlier and keep your stomach from feeling queasy or upset at inopportune times. Sleep schedules can also help reduce potential anxiety because you are making sure your body and mind get adequate rest each night. Although anxiety can make it difficult to sleep, establishing a routine can sometimes help the brain realize when it is supposed to shut down and rest.

Exercise routines are also a good way to keep anxiety down to a minimum. Moving the body during the day promotes overall health by regulating the heart and blood circulation, and producing happy chemicals such as serotonin and dopamine. Exercising also helps to reduce stress and stretch muscles that can become tight and painful with anxiety.

Keeping track of breathing during the day can also help to curb anxiety when it starts sneaking up on someone. Making sure you are taking deep breaths and providing your body with enough oxygen to stay calm can be key when you start to feel symptoms of anxiety. It can even help keep panic attacks from happening if someone can stay calm enough. Refusing to let perfectionistic thoughts rule your brain can also be a tactic to keep anxiety from invading your mind. Part of anxious thoughts include self-criticism and negative self-talk, and if a person can keep these from ruling their decisions and perception, it can be easier to remain calm in the face of anxiety or panic. To do this, you can work on ways to spin negative thoughts into positive sentiments. For example, if you are convinced that you are not good at speaking to others, spin that thought into "I'm a really great listener." Shifting the focus of your thoughts can change your attitude and help you feel more at ease.

Accepting the things you cannot change is another avenue to peace. Anxiety often spurs the need to control your environment and actions so that you can reduce the likelihood of feeling anxious. If you can simply let go of the need to control, however, and accept that the world will be what it is, it can relieve a lot of self-inflicted pressure to make everything perfect. It can be difficult to accept the environment you're in, but with some hard work, it is possible and beneficial.

Anxiety in Public

Unfortunately, anxiety is not restricted to private spaces. It can come on any time, anywhere no matter how inconvenient. For this reason, some people like to have ways that they can deal with anxiety or panic attacks in public without drawing too much attention to their inner struggle. This desire can be especially strong in people who suffer from panic disorder because their attacks are known for their suddenness. Learning how to deal with the warning signs and keep calm in public spaces can help someone to not isolate themselves and be less likely to avoid things.

It can be difficult to manage panic attacks in public because a person is not always in a situation where they can excuse themselves suddenly to deal with their symptoms. They might be in at school or in a meeting at work where their attendance is mandatory. These situations are prime examples of why knowing how to deal with anxiety in public can come in handy. Most people will feel tempted to sulk off into a corner or bathroom stall to deal with their feelings as they come, or to calm themselves down from unforeseen anxiety. Escaping the situation, however, is not actually the best way to handle anxious feelings or thoughts.

First, it is important to remember that panic attacks cannot cause physical harm, despite intense physical symptoms. Yes, they are uncomfortable and scary, but they also are usually fairly short and subside as quickly as they begin. Keeping these rational thoughts in your head can help an attack be less intense and easier to manage.

When a person feels an attack coming on, they should focus more on experiencing the feelings and riding them out than on ignoring or fighting them. If you try to fight off anxious feelings, then the body doesn't have a chance to run its course of adrenaline and panic and will keep pushing for the process to start to finish. So, it can actually help symptoms subside more quickly to just embrace them the first time.

Mindfulness should never be forgotten either, because it is something a person can practice at any time without other people having to know. They can focus on their own breathing instead of the speaker for a moment, or focus on the speaker's wardrobe as a way to force their brain to pick one direction and stick to it. Another interesting tactic that resembles mindfulness is to play scientist. A person can observe their own symptoms as if they were presenting in someone else and take mental notes about severity, duration, and possible causes. This can help them to detach their brain from their feelings and might help them ride out the discomfort.

A third mindful tactic is to use your senses to gather information about the environment you are in. This can be especially helpful if the environment is what triggered your anxiety. Taking a moment to look at everything, listen to the sounds, feel if it's hot or cold, etc., can help you realize that there are no actual threats present and might help to alleviate some worry.

Finally, perhaps the best way to relieve anxiety is to interact with others. Even if this is what is causing your anxiety, talking to other people can help you feel at ease after a while because you realize your fears were all in your head. All it takes is one nice conversation to feel like you are accepted and appreciated.

In some situations, however, it might not be possible for a person to quell their anxiety and they should know when it is time to make an exit instead of pushing forward. Certain places, such as an office, might be especially triggering for someone's anxiety and make them want to leave or quit. Before making this important decision, they should consider their options and not act purely on anxiety because there are ways to cope.

The first thing a person can do is make sure they are aware of their anxious feelings and try to pinpoint the cause of them. This can help them to determine if the job itself is causing them distress or just certain aspects of the environment. Sometimes the root cause is something that is easy to change, such as moving desks to be away from an obnoxious co-worker or eating lunch outside to feel like you are getting away for a moment. Even if it is something not quite as simple, discussing the issue with a boss or supervisor can often lead to positive results.

Another helpful way to deal with anxiety at work is to talk about it. Finding a trusted co-worker or human resources representative to discuss your anxiety with can help you feel like someone will understand if it ever gets bad enough to affect your job. They might even have some advice or solutions to help you with your problems. Even just the act of getting your feelings out in the open can sometimes alleviate some of the stress you felt while keeping them bottled up. Additionally, a lot of people find that hearing their thoughts out loud instead of in their head can help them realize when they are irrational.

It can also be helpful to write down all of the anxious thoughts or feelings you experience at work as a way to get them out of your head and down on paper so you don't feel like you have to carry them around all day. This is also beneficial for being able to see what is going through your mind and possibly identify the thoughts that are not true or a worst-case scenario.

People should also be aware that anxiety can reach a point where it is time to ask for help. If they have tried multiple different coping techniques and nothing seems to be working, then they should consider discussing other options with their boss. Employers are often willing to make accommodations to keep good employees on the payroll and might be surprisingly flexible if they are aware of the situation.

A final strategy a person can use to cope with their anxiety to schedule escapes. This can be a vacation every few months or just a day here and there to stay home and recuperate from the day-to-day stress. Having these scheduled breaks can help someone feel like they don't have to make it at their job every day for the rest of their life, but instead just until their next vacation or day off. If these small breaks are not enough to help the anxiety, then a person might need to consider taking a longer leave from their job. Some companies offer mental health leaves, but others might require an FMLA (Family Medical Leave Act) form stating the individual has an illness that requires them to take time off.

Chapter 8: First Steps

Healing from anxiety can be a long road with a slew of difficult tasks. For some people, this can seem discouraging or intimidating. This is why noticing small accomplishments along the way can help someone stay positive and motivated during their journey to a healthy life. The first step to small successes, however, is accepting anxiety for what it is and how it affects you. Once a person is able to accept the fact that they struggle with anxiety and certain tasks or situations might be more difficult for them, they can start to change their mindset and use anxiety as fuel for a better life.

After a person accepts their anxiety, they can start to consider whether or not they need help to manage it. There are some signs a person can look for in themselves to indicate that it might be time to find someone who can direct them in coping with their anxiety. If they notice these signs, there are many options they can choose from to get the best type of care for their particular situation. Although most people find a mental health professional through a doctor's referral, they can also research professionals on their own and decide who might be best for them.

This chapter discusses how people can turn their anxiety into a positive force in their life by reframing its effects and working with it instead of against it. It also gives tips on what people can look for to know they need help, who can help them with their anxiety, and signs that are making improvement in their journey to health.

Accepting Anxiety

Most people look for ways to fight against their anxiety and might struggle to win that fight their entire lives. Perhaps a more beneficial first step to ending anxiety is to accept its existence and try to reframe its attributes. People can use their anxiety as fuel to accomplish other things in their lives because anxiety itself is not actually bad. Remember that anxiety is a natural response to stimuli and exists to protect us. The way people react to anxiety can be what creates problems and changes in behavior. Changing the way you think about anxiety can change your reaction to its symptoms. For example, if someone starts to feel anxious but uses the adrenaline as fuel to get more tasks completed at work they have just taken the adrenaline the body made for fight or flight and used it for a better purpose.

Achieving a change in mindset can be as simple as changing one thought. Instead of thinking, "Oh my gosh I'm anxious, something terrible is going to happen," a person can think, "Okay, I'm anxious, but that's normal and everything will be okay." This simple change, without even a corresponding action, can turn anxiety from a scary monster into a normal reaction.

Someone can also consider anxiety as their body's way of communicating with them. This can be especially true if the body is responding to one of the HALT triggers explained earlier. If you start to notice you're getting anxious at the same time every day or in similar situations, it might be your body telling you that need a little extra food or sleep, etc., to make it through.

Reframing anxiety can even help people achieve a better work-life balance because this is often a large source of stress for most people. If you can acknowledge that your anxiety stems from the stress of constantly working, then it can be easier to draw the line on where your personal time begins. Making dedicated time to be away from work can ease stress and anxiety and give you a chance to be still and quiet.

A surprisingly common reason for anxiety is people misinterpreting their emotions. For example, feelings of excitement can be similar to those of anxiety and sometimes people get these two emotions confused, especially in new environments. A child might be extremely excited to go to camp for the first time, but his pounding heart and sweaty palms could also make him nervous. Being able to correctly interpret emotions by taking a moment to think them through can help to turn what you might think is anxiety into a much more enjoyable emotion.

People can even use anxiety as a motivator to channel their negative energy into positive activities. If someone with generalized anxiety can learn to channel their anxious feelings into energy to exercise or cleaning their home, they would be successfully establishing healthy routines while working through negative feelings. In addition to anxiety being a motivator, people can use it as fuel to finish projects and operate in high-pressure situations. The body prepares itself to move swiftly when it gets anxious, so a person can use that energy to multitask or power through a time-consuming activity.

Reframing anxiety can help someone take things they are afraid of or things that are stressful and turn them into something powerful and productive. This can help them achieve more, think clearly, and feel less stressed than if they would let their anxiety take control and dominate their thoughts and decisions.

Getting Help

Even though anxiety is something every person will experience at some point in their life, people who experience it frequently tend to feel abnormal or like their brain possibly doesn't work right. These feelings of being an outlier can often keep people from seeking the help they need to manage their anxiety. It can be difficult for them to admit that their anxiety is beyond their control because they often desperately seek to control every aspect of their life as a way of coping. Seeking help can even seem intimidating because they might think that others will judge them or think they are not strong for suffering from a mental illness.

There are many different things that can warn a person it is time for them to get help. The first is if their fear or constant worry has started to interrupt their daily lives. This can mean they are avoiding certain things or struggling to interact with others, but is generally marked in significant changes in their lifestyle due to anxiety. Another common reason to seek help is if anxiety is keeping people from doing things they enjoy. This signals a more severe type of avoidance coping because a person is even afraid to do things that once made them happy.

Fear of speaking up can be another sign that someone should consider seeing a counselor or doctor. If you are afraid to voice your opinions, whether in a group or one-on-one, you might be suffering from social anxiety and getting help quickly can help keep it from developing further.

Sometimes people worry so much that it becomes difficult for them to perform daily functions such as going to work or school, or cleaning the house and cooking food. If anxiety is affecting you to the point where you feel you cannot take care of yourself, seeing a professional can help you take back control of your thoughts and your life. This type of constant worry can also keep someone from completing important or mandatory things, such as attending a work event or leading a meeting. If you find yourself canceling or not attending things that weren't optional, you might want to seek help both for yourself and your job security.

The most important symptom that should receive immediate attention is if someone is feeling detached from their friends, family, and society as a whole. Feeling separated from people who care about you can often lead to worse symptoms and decisions. Counselors and doctors can be the first person someone connects with until they feel comfortable reaching out to people they were once close with.

Someone who is frequently experiencing panic attacks should not suffer alone. This can indicate high levels of anxiety and possibly other issues that need to be addressed. Panic attacks will not necessarily go away on their own, so consider seeking help to alleviate the symptoms and frequency.

Once someone has accepted that they need help managing their anxiety, the next step is finding the right kind of professional. There is a long list of professionals who can help with mental issues, but finding the right type with the right qualifications to meet your needs can require a little research. The number of options might be confusing for some, which can be a good problem to have. There are counselors, psychologists, psychiatrists, therapists, the list goes on. How does a person know who to pick?

Sometimes the best place to start the search is at your primary care doctor's office. Explaining your symptoms to a doctor who knows you is the best way to get an accurate assessment of your risk for an anxiety disorder or if your feelings are due to an underlying medical cause. If your primary doctor thinks counseling or therapy could be beneficial for you, they will typically refer you to another professional they know and trust.

The severity of symptoms and the likelihood of needing medication usually helps a doctor make their decision of who to refer the patient to. If you are not being referred by another doctor, you should also consider these factors; how severe are your symptoms and do you want medication or to manage it on your own? Psychologists are a great option for therapy and typically hold at least a master's degree in psychology. They are trained in therapies such as cognitive behavioral therapy and can help someone talk through their problems and develop plans to alleviate their anxiety. Psychologists cannot, however, prescribe medicine.

Cognitive behavioral therapy is one of the most common types of therapy used to help people who suffer from anxiety. This type of therapy focuses on how a person can modify their thoughts and behaviors to relieve their symptoms. The main thought behind CBT is that a person's thoughts dictate how they view the world and what they might perceive as a threat. By helping someone focus on the positives and create a more realistic view of the world, a psychologist can get them to change negative behaviors and work toward eliminating their anxiety.

If a psychologist believes medication might help a patient, and the patient is in agreement, they will usually refer them to a psychiatrist. A psychiatrist is a medical doctor who studied psychology and is trained in both therapy and medicine. They can act as a therapist and prescribe medication to patients to help them better manage their symptoms. Sometimes pairing medicine with therapy is the best option for people suffering from intense symptoms. Having one doctor in charge of both aspects of your care can also help to streamline effectiveness and not end up on a medicine that doesn't work or makes you feel worse.

An alternative to psychiatrists is a psychiatric nurse practitioner. These professionals can do all the same things as psychiatrists — see patients and prescribe medicine — but earned a nursing degree instead of a doctoral degree. These professionals typically work under the supervision of a doctor, but can have their own practices within that scope.

It can take a long time for someone to completely heal from having anxiety and learn to deal with their symptoms in a healthy way. On this journey, however, there are some milestones they can look to accomplish as a way of measuring progress. Sometimes noticing these small victories can help a person stay on track to success.

A person can tell their anxiety is improving if they notice themselves starting to interact more with other people. Along with this, they might also stop avoiding social situations as much as in the past and possibly even begin to seek out other people.

This can be a great sign that social anxiety is being alleviated and a person is able to work through their fears and talk to others despite it.

Some people who begin taking charge of their anxiety also notice some of their energy coming back during the process. Worry and stress can sap most of someone's energy during the day to the point they might not want to do anything by the time they get home. Regaining some of it is a sign that you are less worried and your body can handle more of other things.

When anxiety starts to fade away, a person will usually notice themselves feeling happier. They might smile more, hear their own laugh for the first time in months, or generally appreciate life more than when they were anxious. Allowing yourself to be happy is a key step in healing and a good indicator that you are making progress. Along with this change in demeanor might also be the act of choosing happier clothes. Someone making progress in their therapy might start choosing more colorful clothes that make them stand out and get noticed. This can be a subconscious way of inviting others to interact with them and marks a positive improvement in anxiety levels.

Eating can be an issue for some people with anxiety, as the symptoms can cause a lack of appetite or lead to binge eating. As a person heals, however, they might notice their eating habits returning to normal and their food decisions improving.

Accomplishing lists and to-dos can be another sign that a person is making headway in their efforts. These tasks can be difficult for someone with anxiety to manage when they are plagued with worry and doubt, but if they find themselves completing them with ease it usually means they are handling their symptoms more effectively.

Anxiety and stress can make a person tense and tighten muscles throughout their body. Once they learn to relax, especially through yoga or muscle relaxation techniques, they can usually feel their muscles start to unwind and experience less pain due to tightness and stress.

As people start to get a grip on their struggles, they might also notice themselves doing a better job at keeping their home clean and neat if they prefer it that way. This can be a good sign that a person's anxiety has let up enough for it not to consume all of their thoughts.

Finally, a great sign and benefit of anxiety leaving a person's mind is when they can sleep through the night. If you can make it through the night without interruptions or tossing and turning, it can be a sign that your mind is learning how to be quiet and calm.

Chapter 9: The Road to Healing

Healing is a unique experience for everyone who goes through it. For some, it is quick, for others lengthy, and still others fall somewhere in between. It has to do with the severity of symptoms, willingness to change, and time spent working on reaching goals. Some people are able to achieve their happy ending on their own, by reading books like this one or doing their own research and finding techniques that help them manage their anxiety and continue living a normal life. Others might decide they need a little help to make it through a particularly difficult time, and that's okay too.

There are a number of tricks to manage anxiety and reduce the frequency of panic attacks, and everyone has their own tactic that works best for them. The key to these tips and tricks is to continue trying different ones until a person finds one that works. There are natural remedies such as essential oils, relaxation techniques such as deep breathing, and even cognitive behavioral therapy exercises that can be found online. Not each one of these will work for everyone, though, and people should not be discouraged if they try one method and it doesn't work for them.

Overcoming fears can be the most difficult part of taking charge of anxiety, but it is also the most important. Avoiding things a person is afraid of can only make those things seem scarier, but facing them head-on can often take away the mystery and fear. Sometimes to achieve this, a person will employ the help of a doctor or counselor to assist them with developing an action plan and staying on track. This can also help a person more accurately measure their progress and receive feedback from another informed person. This chapter discusses ways a person can manage their anxiety, reduce the frequency of panic attacks, overcome their fears, and ensure their therapy is working for them.

Managing Symptoms

Learning to manage anxiety can be difficult and uncomfortable. It might mean going against all of the signals your brain is sending to face a fear that seems insurmountable. It is important to remember during this time that working with your doctor to learn new coping skills can be the best and fastest way to start effectively fighting off your anxiety.

The first trick is to learn how to embrace uncertainty. Anxiety can often make someone afraid of the parts of life they don't understand or situations they can't control. Learning to accept that not all things are within your power to manipulate and predict can help you release some of the stress that comes from trying to shape your environment to your needs. Part of embracing uncertainty is being able to recognize when you are obsessing over one thought or worry. Sometimes it can be difficult for anxious people to solve problems or work through logical situations because an anxious thought is spinning around in their brain and dominating their thought process. If they can learn to stop and recognize these thoughts, it can be easier to regain control of their mind and accept that some things are unknown.

Perhaps the best way to learn and practice these skills is by using mindfulness techniques. Being mindful of yourself and your thoughts can make it much easier to notice when they start erring toward anxiety and away from calm and rational. This way, you can take back control of your thoughts before they spiral too far down the wrong path. These techniques can also reduce worry and increase willpower. If a person is able to tap into their body's needs at any time, it can relax their sense of uncertainty and give them a feeling that they are back in control. These exercises can include setting intentions at the beginning of each day, meditating, going for a walk, or simply looking up at the sky to notice all the things that would normally pass by without a second glance. People can also make a point to put their phone down for an extended period of time to make time to take care of themselves and not have to worry about others. If they want to take this exercise to the next level, they can even leave their phone at home when they go out to experience a release from technology.

One tactic commonly used in cognitive behavioral therapy is to encourage people to realize when their thoughts are distorted.

This can be in any number of ways such as underestimating their own abilities, predicting negative outcomes, or catastrophizing. If you can start to identify these thoughts for what they are, it is easier to resist the temptation to cave to them and continue with calmness.

It is also important for people to remember that most therapies will not give results right away. They take hard work and dedication to start yielding benefits. Typically, cognitive behavioral therapy takes about 12 to 16 weeks before a person will start seeing marked improvement in their symptoms.

Along with managing their anxiety, a person can also work to reduce the frequency of their panic attacks. Learning to manage panic can be just as stressful as facing fears with anxiety, but once a person can learn to take control of their mind and not be intimidated by their symptoms, having a panic attack might not be the terrible thing it once was.

The first step a person can take to reduce their panic attacks is to make sure they are sticking with the treatment plan their doctor devised with them. It can be difficult to face things alone once you leave the doctor's office, but making sure you are practicing the techniques he or she teaches you is imperative to success. Sometimes joining a support group can help you to follow through with the action plan. People often find that having a group of others who truly understand and experience the same problems can help them see their issues from a different perspective or find the support they need to continue working toward their goal.

Just like people with anxiety, people who experience frequent panic attacks should limit or avoid exposure to stimulants and depressants such as caffeine, drugs, and alcohol. These substances can make it more difficult to deal with feelings and recognize what your triggers are, so it is best to keep them out of a regular routine.

Stress management tactics are another helpful way to get a grip on panic attacks. People can focus on turning their negative thoughts into positive actions; this might take a little more skill than if someone was dealing with anxiety alone because of the suddenness of panicked thoughts. They can also focus on being assertive instead of aggressive when they are feeling irritated by exercising regularly, and making a schedule to effectively manage their time and tasks.

Relaxation techniques also work equally well for managing panic attacks as with anxiety. Things such as yoga, deep breathing, and muscle relaxation can help the body to calm down even in the face of panicked thoughts or physical symptoms. Making sure you get enough sleep at night is another way to relax the body. Having a schedule for bedtime and wake up times can be incredibly helpful to calm the body because it has a predictable schedule.

If these milder approaches are not doing the trick, sometimes exposure therapy can be the best option for a person to face their fears and decrease the likelihood of a panic attack. This type of therapy involves a person subjecting themselves to the very thing that they are afraid will incite an attack. Typically, this process can be painful the first few times, but after a while, the person will realize the situation does not pose any threat and there is no reason to feel anxious or panicked.

Some people opt for home remedies to treat panic attacks, especially at their onset. Inhaling lavender essential oils, or putting some in a diffuser, is possibly the most common way people can ease their worry homeopathically. Lavender is known for its calming effects and ability to relax the nervous system.

Moving Forward

An important part of the healing process when someone is overcoming anxiety and panic attacks is to confront their fears. When a person continually avoids things that cause them anxiety, it can cement the fear in their brain and make it more and more intense as time goes on. In order to face their fears, however, a person needs to understand how their brain reacts in scary situations so they can start to identify their triggers and responses. Once they know these two things, staying ahead of the curve can become much easier and the odds of successfully controlling anxiety can increase.

The first step is to refuse to be afraid of feeling fear. Sometimes the suggestions of fear, such as a trailer for a horror movie, can be enough to get someone's anxiety moving. You can't necessarily avoid commercials for horror movies, though, so a person has to learn that the suggestion of fear and fear itself are two different things. Avoidance can keep a person from doing a number of things in their life, even things they used to enjoy. Fear can be a powerful motivator to stay away from something, but if a person can take a deep breath and acknowledge that it might not spark fear then they could have a better chance of confronting it without anxiety.

Exposure therapy usually comes into play after this first step. A person should pick one of their fears that they are motivated to overcome and talk to their doctor about steps to safely expose themselves and become desensitized. Usually, the first time someone practices exposure will be the longest exercise because the trick to this therapy is remaining exposed to the stimulus until the person is able to calm down and feel comfortable. The exercise is repeated over and over once a week or every few days until the person no longer feels afraid of the stimulus. For example, if someone is agoraphobic, their doctor might have someone take them to a grocery store near their home. They would walk around the store until they felt at ease with being in public and around others. This type of therapy helps to teach the brain that what it perceives as a threat is not actually dangerous and the negative outcome it predicted is not real.

People can also overcome their fears by focusing on the positive things in life. You can take a piece of paper and write down all the things you are grateful for to shift your focus onto happiness. It can also be a great reminder of the different people and reasons that make fighting off anxiety, worth it. Using humor is also an effective way to lessen anxiety and forget your fears. If someone starts to feel worried, they can make up the most out-of-this-world worst-case scenario, such as aliens landing at the dinner party and there not being enough food to serve all of them, to help them realize how silly some of their worries really are. Learning to appreciate this sense of humor and not taking yourself too seriously can help reduce stress and anxiety simultaneously.

Even when a person is dedicated to facing their fears and reducing their anxiety, it can still be difficult to do alone. Deciding to start therapy can be a major decision for some people and once they start, they might not feel like they are making any progress in the beginning. Trusting a therapist can take time, but they are there to support and help you. A therapist can monitor someone's successes and progress and keep them motivated to continue with treatment. Having this consistent, unbiased support can help a person remember that therapy takes time and effort to work.

Most therapists who utilize cognitive behavioral therapy are frequently checking in with their patients and discussing their symptoms, goals, and behaviors. By assessing the person's emotional state and progress, they are able to keep them on track toward achieving their long and short-term goals. This is also how the therapist can make sure that the person is enacting their plan and working on changing their thoughts and behaviors.

If you ever feel concerned that you are not making enough progress while in therapy, you can always ask your doctor to give their opinion. They might discuss with you the steps you've taken in the right direction and things they think might still be holding you back. Most likely, however, they will tell you not to worry because everyone heals at different speeds and as long as you are putting in the work you will get the results.

Having a positive relationship with your doctor can also help you feel like you are making progress because it develops trust. It also helps you to open up and let them know all of your symptoms and feelings so together you can form a comprehensive, realistic action plan that targets them all. When a more detailed action plan can be created, faster results are more likely to occur because the doctor can target very specific things with realistic expectations. This can also help someone to trust their doctor more because they see the results they hoped for and are acknowledging that the hard work is paying off.

Sometimes people want to be able to gauge their success on their own, though, to be able to make their own progress chart. To accomplish this, the first thing you can do is ask yourself how your mood has been impacted by therapy. Has it generally improved, stayed the same, or is it getting worse? If your mood is improving, that can be a good sign that you are improving in small ways also. Another question to ask yourself is if your behaviors have changed since starting therapy. This question can sometimes take a little more self-examination than the first, but can be another good way to score your progress. A helpful way to measure this is to keep a journal of your reactions to anxious situations so you can see if there are any marked improvements over time.

Finally, a person can also consider whether or not they are solving problems on their own. If they are, this can also indicate that they are working on achieving both their short- and long-term goals.

Chapter 10: Meditation to Calm the Mind

Meditation is a common exercise people use to quiet their minds and reduce stress. It has worked wonders for so many people, possibly because there are so many different types and techniques, which makes it easy for someone to find a kind of meditation that works for them. From mindfulness practices to yoga and positive self-talk, meditation can form to a person's individual needs and help them to find calmness and peace-of-mind they might be missing while dealing with their symptoms. It can be difficult to get into at first, but once a person masters meditating they often see marked improvements in their mood and stress levels.

Yoga is a common exercise that people might not always associate with meditating, but it was created by ancient religions as a way to do just that. The different yoga practices all focus on making the mind aware of the body as it stretches and strengthens the muscles. It focuses on deep breathing to relax a person so they can achieve a deeper stretch and have a more peaceful experience. Many yoga classes even directly incorporate meditation into the poses by instructing people to listen to their breathing and focus on how it affects their bodies.

Meditating can be a simple way to reduce stress, quiet the mind, and become more focused during the day. It can reduce physical pain by working to lower stress hormones and responses in the body so a person feels both mentally and physically healthier. This chapter explores common meditation practices, how yoga can reduce stress, all the ways meditation can help someone reduce anxiety, and directions on how to use meditation effectively in your life.

Common Practices

Meditation can be a great way to reduce stress and limit the effects of anxiety. It is also useful because it can be practiced at any time and in any place, making it a great tool for people who experience symptoms in public. Teaching your mind to calm down and focus can not only reduce anxiety, but also stress and worry as well. Meditation is usually considered complementary to therapy because it can help a person get into the right mindset to begin examining themselves and their symptoms. It can also help them remain calm during difficult exercises such as confronting fears or identifying triggers.

The point of meditation is to focus the mind on something simple instead of letting negative thoughts turn into messy knotted bunches in your brain. Meditation takes people through exercises where they can start to pull at the strings of these knots and slowly untangle them until they feel at peace again. There are a number of different meditation practices you can use, including some physical activities and some resting mental activities, that can help you to calm down and focus. Some people prefer to do activities where they sit still and focus, and others like the distraction of moving during their meditation.

Guided meditation is one type of sedentary meditation that can be especially helpful for beginners. In this type, a person's voice moves you through meditation by telling you what to focus on and what to do with your body. It can help people with no meditation experience learn the basics and find a natural rhythm that they can later keep on their own. Mantra meditation is similar to this tactic, but it does not involve another person. The meditator finds a word or phrase that helps them to calm down and then repeats it during their meditation and lets the words become their focus.

Mindfulness meditation is a way to employ two calming techniques at once and engage all of your senses. It focuses on increasing awareness of your surroundings and your body as a means of accepting the world you live in for what it is. This type of meditation can also help people to practice living in the moment instead of worrying about the past or future. People typically focus on their body, such as the rhythm of their breathing and the deepness of their breath, how their muscles feel when they take in air and release it. When an anxious thought pops into your head during meditation, this type suggests you acknowledge its existence and then let it go; don't waste time or energy entertaining all its possibilities.

More physical versions of meditation include Tai Chi and yoga. Tai Chi focuses on slow, deliberate movements while taking purposeful breaths. It can help people learn how to breathe during a physical response to anxiety, teach calmness, and improve balance. Yoga can be a little more intense than Tai Chi, depending on what type of practice a person is attempting. It focuses on listening to the body and responding to its needs through a series of poses intended to stretch and release different muscles. Yoga often ends with a few minutes to lie in silence and feel the muscles of your body and your breathing work together to support you.

How it Helps

Yoga combines the three main relaxation techniques that people with anxiety and panic disorders frequently utilize: deep breathing, muscle relaxation, and visualization. These three things create a stress-free, peace-inducing atmosphere that makes it easy to let go of stress and worry. Yoga has been known to help people reduce stress, lower blood pressure, and lower heart rate by pairing exercise with meditation. Its anxious roots have always focused on finding inner peace and becoming one with the earth, which can help some people to feel more connected to their environment instead of afraid of it.

Because yoga is a physical activity, it can help promote mindfulness and relieve some of the physical symptoms of anxiety. Often, people who are anxious suffer from stiff or sore muscles from holding tension in their body for prolonged periods of time. Yoga can help them stretch those muscles and relieve some of the tension they feel on a daily basis.

The goal of yoga is to stretch, lengthen, and strengthen muscles as a form of meditation. The physical response to different poses gives a person something to focus on instead of the thoughts running through their head. It can help some people feel more in touch with their bodies and become more aware of its signals. It is a good outlet for someone who wants a more intense meditative work out than Tai Chi or walking because they can definitely work up a sweat doing yoga. Finding the right type for their skill level and based on desired results can also be helpful to find one that gives them just enough exercise to feel like they've accomplished something.

Joining a yoga class can also be a great way to meet new people and interact with someone every day. This can be great for people who are trying not to withdraw from others and push their social boundaries each week. During the class, they can quiet their mind enough to build up the courage to speak to someone after the lesson is over.

There are many different types of yoga that could be beneficial for a beginner, such as Hatha or Asana yoga. Hatha yoga has a slower pace than most practices and easier movements. It is often focused a little more on meditating and being aware of the body than deeply stretching muscles. Asana yoga is a bit more fast-paced and focuses on movement and stretching a little more than meditation, but usually ends with time to meditate and reflect on the openness of your muscles after practice.

Beginners can sometimes be intimidated if they walk into a yoga class and do not know what to expect. All types of yoga are made up of a sequence of poses that are combined to move your body through a logical pattern of stretching. They all come together to help release tension and relax the muscles while also promoting flexibility and strength. Poses can range from lying on the floor to standing on one leg with arms outstretched. Yoga can help people with a variety of chronic conditions such as anxiety, panic disorder, or illnesses that cause significant pain.

Meditation can help both mental and physical health by giving people a sense of balance, calm, and inner peace. These things can carry throughout their day beyond their meditation session to help them feel calm and in control. Sometimes this feeling alone is enough to help someone cope with their anxiety. It can also help people to clear their minds of the clutter and stress they carry with them during the day. Having a blank slate to start the day with can make the onslaught of tasks feel much more manageable and keep a person from feeling like they are overwhelmed or out of control.

Taking time to meditate can also help someone see a new perspective about something they were maybe obsessing over or worrying about. Sometimes being able to see a problem in a new light can help you feel less anxious about it and understand it better. If a person can take the time during the day to look for new ways to view their anxiety, it can make it easier to deal with when it flares up.

Meditation even promotes an increased self-awareness, which can help some people focus on the present during the day. Being able to keep the mind in the present moment and not wander into regrets of the past or possibilities of the future, can be an incredibly effective way for people to avoid anxiety panic attacks. Along with this awareness can come patience, tolerance, imagination, and creativity. All of these qualities can encourage a person to be kinder to themselves and others and possibly even be more productive at work because their brains are free to explore, unencumbered by negative thoughts.

Mental peace can sometimes even aid in physical recovery, especially those illnesses that are worsened by stress. By calming people, meditation can help to reduce inflammation in the body that is caused by stress hormones. Reducing this internal inflammation can often relieve a considerable amount of pain for people. Aside from pain, research suggests meditating can help people who suffer from a wide range of symptoms including, asthma, heart disease, high blood pressure, sleep problems, and headaches. It could be because all of these symptoms can be worsened by stress and once that is alleviated the symptoms are alleviated too.

In addition to mental and physical health, meditating can even help someone lengthen their attention span. This can be extremely helpful both at work and in school, especially if a person suffers from an attention disorder or has trouble focusing their mind on the conversation and not on their own anxiety. It can also help older adults who are starting to suffer from memory loss due to their age. This is because when a person improves their attention span and their clarity of mind, it can help the brain retain characteristics of a younger person such as holding on to and being able to recall memories.

Finally, perhaps the best benefit of meditating is that people don't have to do it at home. If you are anxious before a big meeting, take a moment at your desk to meditate and focus on your breathing until you feel you have calmed down enough to step into the boardroom. You don't have to wait for an appointment or have someone guide you, meditation is always available when you need it.

Meditation can be difficult to get used to, especially if your brain is used to traveling a mile a minute. Racing thoughts can be difficult to quiet without a little practice, so people should remember that their first couple of attempts to meditate might not go as seamlessly as they hoped for.

The key to effective meditation can be to find a time in your day where it fits rather seamlessly. This can help you avoid stressing about when you will ever find time to meditate, which is the opposite of the exercise's goal. If you are a morning person, you might want to wake up a few minutes early to sit in peace for a moment before starting your daily routine. If you know you always have extra time on your lunch break, that might be a good time to sneak in five minutes of meditation. Even if you are only doing it in the moments before you fall asleep at night, finding any time to quiet your mind during the day can be beneficial to managing anxiety.

Some people might feel confused about how long they are supposed to meditate for. This factor depends entirely on them and how much time they have during the day to dedicate to meditation, how long they would like to meditate for, and what are their attitudes toward the exercise. For people who are meditating for the first time, a good goal is to try the practice for 5 to 10 minutes every day. If this seems too long, or you are having trouble staying focused for the entire time, then feel free to shorten it to a duration you are comfortable with. Once you are used to meditating for a certain amount of time, if you would like to increase the duration, simply add one minute at a time and let yourself gradually get used to the new limit. A person should never increase their time until they are able to be still and calm for the entire duration of their meditation without issue.

Before sitting down to meditate, a person should first consider what makes them happy and what they want to visualize during their exercise. This can be in the form of a mantra or a mental picture that helps the person to quiet their mind and feel relaxed.

After they establish this, they can consider their goals and what they are hoping to get out of meditating to set their intentions for the session.

One of the most important lessons someone can learn from meditation is patience. It teaches people to be calm and still in the presence of nothingness and that results come in due time. This can sometimes make people uncomfortable at first because society has become so skilled at bombarding people with information all the time, but it is worth learning for inner peace.

It typically takes a few weeks for someone to start noticing the results of their new meditation habit, as long as they are keeping it in their regular routine. The best way to do this is to make it part of a daily ritual such as brushing your teeth or taking a shower. If you can work-in meditation as a mandatory task each day, you are more likely to reap its benefits.

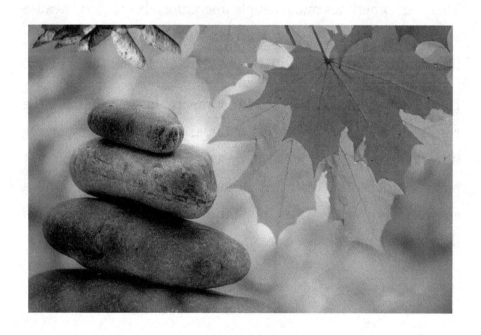

Conclusion

Even though anxiety can be difficult to manage, people should not feel like they have to struggle with it forever. The first step to recovery is often acknowledging its many symptoms such as sweating, trembling, a racing heart, and nervousness. Making efforts not to let anxious thoughts control your day and decisions can be difficult, but it can help to keep you from having panic attacks. Learning how to ride out the symptoms of anxiety and panic takes a lot of practice and it is important not to get discouraged or start avoiding situations due to anxiety.

Getting Help

Sometimes dealing with anxiety can be too much for someone to handle without professional help. It can be difficult to admit what seems like defeat and call a doctor, but it can be the best way for people with severe symptoms to find relief. There is a wide array of options to choose from when picking a doctor. If a person is too overwhelmed by their choices, they can always go to their primary care doctor who can then refer them to a trusted psychologist or counselor. After establishing a relationship with the therapist, you can then work on establishing trust and working toward a long-term goal with milestones along the way.

Meditation

Therapists will sometimes recommend meditation as a supplement to other activities that help alleviate anxiety. Exercises such as mindfulness and yoga can help someone take a step back from their negative thoughts and find a moment to calm themselves down. This can give them a chance to rationally work through their anxious thoughts and calm their body before panic sets in. The key to reaping the benefits of meditation is to do it regularly and focus on releasing negative thoughts and replace them with positive attitudes.

References

Amatenstein, S. (n.d.). Facing Your Fears: Tips to Overcoming
Anxiety and Phobias. Retrieved from:
https://www.psycom.net/facing-your-fear

Anxiety and Depression Association of America. (n.d.). Facts
and Statistics. Retrieved from: https://adaa.org/about-
adaa/press-room/facts-statistics

Anxiety and Depression Association of America. (n.d.). Helpful
Guide to Different Therapy Options. Retrieved from:
https://adaa.org/finding-help/treatment/therapy

Anxiety and Depression Association of America. (n.d.). Panic
Disorder. Retrieved from: https://adaa.org/understanding-
anxiety/panic-disorder

Anxiety and Depression Association of America. (n.d.). Tips.
Retrieved from: https://adaa.org/tips

Anxiety and Depression Association of America. (n.d.).
Understanding Anxiety. Retrieved from:
https://adaa.org/understanding-anxiety/panic-disorder-
agoraphobia/symptoms

Anxiety Disorders. (n.d.). Retrieved from:
https://www.nami.org/learn-more/mental-health-
conditions/anxiety-disorders

Barthel, A., Hay, A., Hofmann, S. (n.d.). Panic Attacks and Panic Disorder: Symptoms, Treatment, Causes, and Coping Strategies. Retrieved from: https://www.anxiety.org/panic-disorder-panic-attacks#treatment-options

Beck, J. (2015). How to Know if Therapy is Working. Retrieved from: https://beckinstitute.org/how-to-know-if-therapy-is-working/

Boomsma, D., Burri, A., Davies, M., Hettema, J., Jansen, R., Lee, M., Spector, T., Trzaskowski, M., Verdi, S. (2015). Generalized Anxiety Disorder — A Twin Study of Genetic Architecture, Genome-Wide Association and Differential Gene Expression. Retrieved from: https://www.ncbi.nlm.nih.gov/pmc/articles/PMC4537268/

Boyes, A. (2012). Cognitive Behavioral Skills You'll Need to Beat Anxiety. Retrieved from: https://www.psychologytoday.com/us/blog/in-practice/201212/cognitive-behavioral-skills-youll-need-beat-anxiety

Brook, C., Schmidt, L. (2008). Social Anxiety Disorder: A Review of Environmental Risk Factors. Retrieved from: https://www.ncbi.nlm.nih.gov/pmc/articles/PMC2515922/

Carter, S., Jovanovic, T., Keller, J., Lott, A., Michopoulos, V., Ogbonmwan, Y., Rooij, S., Stenson, A., Stevens, J. (n.d.). What is Anxiety? Retrieved from: https://www.anxiety.org/what-is-anxiety

Causes, Signs, and Effects of Panic Disorder. (n.d.). Retrieved from: https://www.belmontbehavioral.com/disorders/panic/causes-effects/

Cherney, K. (2018). Effects of Anxiety on the Body. Retrieved from: https://www.healthline.com/health/anxiety/effects-on-body#1

Cirino, E. (2016). Everything You Need to Know About Anxiety. Retrieved from: https://www.healthline.com/health/anxiety-symptoms

Crawford, J. (2018). How Can You Stop a Panic Attack? Retrieved from: https://www.medicalnewstoday.com/articles/321510.php

Cuncic, A. (2019). How to Accept and Stop Controlling Your Social Anxiety. Retrieved from: https://www.verywellmind.com/how-to-accept-social-anxiety-3024895

Dix, M. (n.d.). How Long Should You Meditate to Get Real Results? Retrieved from: https://www.doyouyoga.com/how-long-should-you-meditate-to-get-real-results/

Domschke, K., Gottschalk, M. (2017). Genetics of Generalized Anxiety Disorder and Related Traits. Retrieved from: https://www.ncbi.nlm.nih.gov/pmc/articles/PMC5573560/

Domschke, K., Gottschalk, M. (2016). Novel Developments in Genetic and Epigenetic Mechanisms of Anxiety. Retrieved from: https://www.ncbi.nlm.nih.gov/pubmed/26575296

Felman, A. (2018). What Causes Anxiety? Retrieved from: https://www.medicalnewstoday.com/articles/323456.php

Ferguson, S. (2019). Is Anxiety Genetic? Retrieved from: https://www.healthline.com/health/mental-health/is-anxiety-genetic

Ferreira, M. (2017). Fourteen Mindfulness Tricks to Reduce Anxiety. Retrieved from: https://www.healthline.com/health/mindfulness-tricks-to-reduce-anxiety#1

Generalized Anxiety Disorder. (n.d.). Retrieved from: https://www.helpguide.org/articles/anxiety/generalized-anxiety-disorder-gad.htm

Goldacre, M., Hawton, K., Ross, J., Seminog, O., Singhal, A. (2014). Risk of Self-Harm and Suicide in People with Specific Psychiatric and Physical Disorders: Comparisons Between Disorders Using English National Record Linkage. Retrieved from: https://www.ncbi.nlm.nih.gov/pmc/articles/PMC4023515/

Gotter, A. (2018). Eleven Ways to Stop a Panic Attack. Retrieved from: https://www.healthline.com/health/how-to-stop-a-panic-attack#focus-object

Greenstein, L. (2018). What to Do If Your Workplace is Anxiety-Inducing. Retrieved from: https://www.nami.org/Blogs/NAMI-Blog/February-2018/What-To-Do-if-Your-Workplace-is-Anxiety-Inducing

Griswold, D. (2018). Unusual Ways That Anxiety Affects Behavior. Retrieved from: https://www.calmclinic.com/anxiety/symptoms/behavior

Haas, S. (2018). Help for Anxiety: Facing Your Fears Will Heal Your Brain. Retrieved from: psychologytoday.com/us/blog/prescriptions-life/201808/help-anxiety-facing-your-fears-will-heal-your-brain

Harvard Health Publishing. (2019). Generalized Anxiety Disorder. Retrieved from: https://www.health.harvard.edu/mind-and-mood/generalized-anxiety-disorder

Holland, K. (2018). Everything You Need to Know About Anxiety. Retrieved from: https://www.healthline.com/health/anxiety

Holland, K. (2018). What Triggers Anxiety? Eleven Causes That May Surprise You. Retrieved from: https://www.healthline.com/health/anxiety/anxiety-triggers

Jacofsky, M., Khemlani-Patel, S., Neziroglu, F., Santos, M. (n.d.). The Symptoms of Anxiety. Retrieved from: https://www.gracepointwellness.org/1-anxiety-disorders/article/38467-the-symptoms-of-anxiety

Legg, T. (2016). Doctors Who Treat Anxiety. Retrieved from: https://www.healthline.com/health/anxiety-doctors

Li, P., Stamatakis, J. (2011). What Happens in the Brain When We Experience a Panic Attack? Retrieved from: https://www.scientificamerican.com/article/what-happens-in-the-brain-when-we-experience/

Lindberg, S. (2018). Five Ways Accepting Your Anxiety Can Make You More Powerful. Retrieved from: https://www.healthline.com/health/how-anxiety-can-make-you-more-powerful#1

Mayo Clinic. (n.d.). Meditation: A Simple, Fast Way to Reduce Stress. Retrieved from: https://www.mayoclinic.org/tests-procedures/meditation/in-depth/meditation/art-20045858

Mayo Clinic. (n.d.). Panic Attacks and Panic Disorder. Retrieved from: https://www.mayoclinic.org/diseases-conditions/panic-attacks/symptoms-causes/syc-20376021

Mayo Clinic. (n.d.). Social Anxiety Disorder (Social Phobia). Retrieved from: https://www.mayoclinic.org/diseases-conditions/social-anxiety-disorder/symptoms-causes/syc-20353561

Meditation FAQs. (n.d.). Retrieved from:
https://siyli.org/resources/how-often-when-meditate

Meek, W. (2019). Generalized Anxiety Disorder: Causes and
Risk Factors. Retrieved from:
https://www.verywellmind.com/gad-causes-risk-factors-
1392982

Morris-Rosendahl, D. (2002). Are There Anxious Genes?
Retrieved from:
https://www.ncbi.nlm.nih.gov/pmc/articles/PMC3181683/

Mulpeter, K. (2016). These Groups are Most at Risk for Anxiety
Disorders. Retrieved from:
https://www.health.com/anxiety/anxiety-disorders-women

Panic Attacks and Panic Disorder. (n.d.). Retrieved from:
https://www.helpguide.org/articles/anxiety/panic-attacks-
and-panic-disorders.htm

Panicking in Public? Five Surprising Tips for Getting Through
and Attack. (2018). Retrieved from:
https://health.clevelandclinic.org/panicking-in-public-5-
surprising-tips-for-getting-through-an-attack/

Quinn, H. (2017). 47 Little Signs You're Recovering From
Anxiety. Retrieved from:
https://themighty.com/2017/07/little-signs-recovering-
anxiety/

Risk Factors for Generalized Anxiety Disorder. (n.d.). Retrieved from: https://www.winchesterhospital.org/health-library/article?id=19481

Rodriguez, D. (2009). How to Handle Panic Attacks. Retrieved from: https://www.everydayhealth.com/anxiety/how-to-handle-panic-attacks.aspx

Schlossberg, M. (2017). Thirteen Signs It's Time to Get Help for Your Anxiety. Retrieved from: https://www.redbookmag.com/body/mental-health/g13445934/help-for-anxiety/

Signs and Symptoms of Anxiety. (n.d.). Retrieved from: https://www.valleybehavioral.com/anxiety/signs-symptoms-causes/

Star, K. (2019). How Yoga Can Help Ease Anxiety and Panic Disorder Symptoms. Retrieved from: https://www.verywellmind.com/yoga-for-panic-disorder-2584114

Star, K. (2019). What Does a Panic Attack Feel Like? Retrieved from: https://www.verywellmind.com/panic-attack-basics-2583945

Stress Management. (n.d.). Retrieved from: https://www.webmd.com/balance/stress-management/stress-management

Thorpe, M. (2017). Twelve Science-Based Benefits of Meditation. Retrieved from: https://www.healthline.com/nutrition/12-benefits-of-meditation#section1

Therapy for Anxiety Disorders. (n.d.). Retrieved from: https://www.helpguide.org/articles/anxiety/therapy-for-anxiety-disorders.htm

Vann, M. (2015). Is Anxiety Hereditary? Retrieved from: https://www.everydayhealth.com/news/is-anxiety-hereditary/

WebMD. (2019). Ways to Stop a Panic Attack. Retrieved from: https://www.webmd.com/anxiety-panic/ss/slideshow-ways-to-stop-panic-attack

What Happens During a Panic Attack? (n.d.). Retrieved from: https://www.webmd.com/anxiety-panic/panic-attack-happening#1

What You Should Know About the Link Between Anxiety and Self-Harm. (2019). Retrieved from: https://www.goodtherapy.org/blog/what-you-should-know-about-the-link-between-anxiety-self-harm-0207197

CPSIA information can be obtained
at www.ICGtesting.com
Printed in the USA
BVHW041331231020
591690BV00011B/798